by Neil B. Brahe, DDS

Originally published anonymously in 1962
by Project D, the publishing
imprint of Neil B. Brahe, DDS,
of Appleton, Wisconsin.

This edition published in 2016 by
About Comics, Camarillo, California.

Inquiries? Want a custom cover edition?
Email *questions@aboutcomics.com*

THE ONLY SERIOUS THOUGHT IN THIS BOOK:

THIS LITTLE GEM WAS PRODUCED WITH ONE
THOUGHT IN MIND. THAT MY HARD WORKING
COLLEAGUES MAY, IN THE HEAT OF A BUSY DAY,
SIT BACK AND CHUCKLE..

I HAVE FOUND THROUGH THE YEARS THAT A
LAUGH AT OURSELVES IS THE VERY BEST KIND..

IF IT WILL CUT THE CORONARY RATE BY ONE-MILLIONTH
OF ONE PERCENT IT WILL HAVE BEEN WORTH WHILE..

ANY RESEMBLANCE TO ANYONE EXCEPT MYSELF
IS AN ARTIFACT..

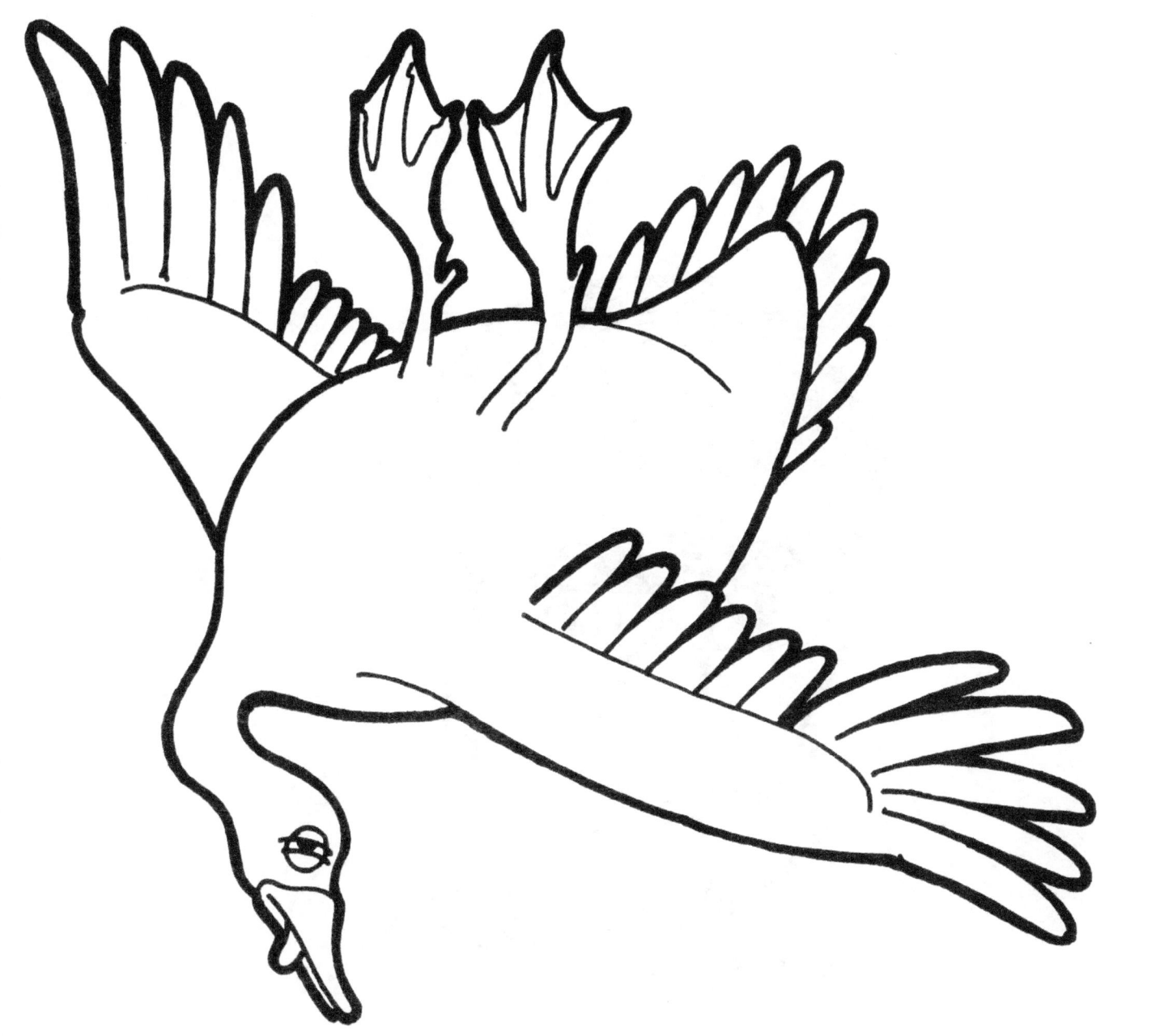

THIS IS A **DEAD DUCK** · AND IF THE DENTAL SOCIETY·
ANY HYGENIST · SUPPLY MAN · OR ANY OF MY
FORMER ASSISTANTS EVER FIND OUT WHO I AM·
THAT'S EXACTLY WHAT I'LL BE · THEREFORE I
PREFER ANONIMITY···

NO DEDICATIONS
NO ONE WANTS ANY PART OF IT!

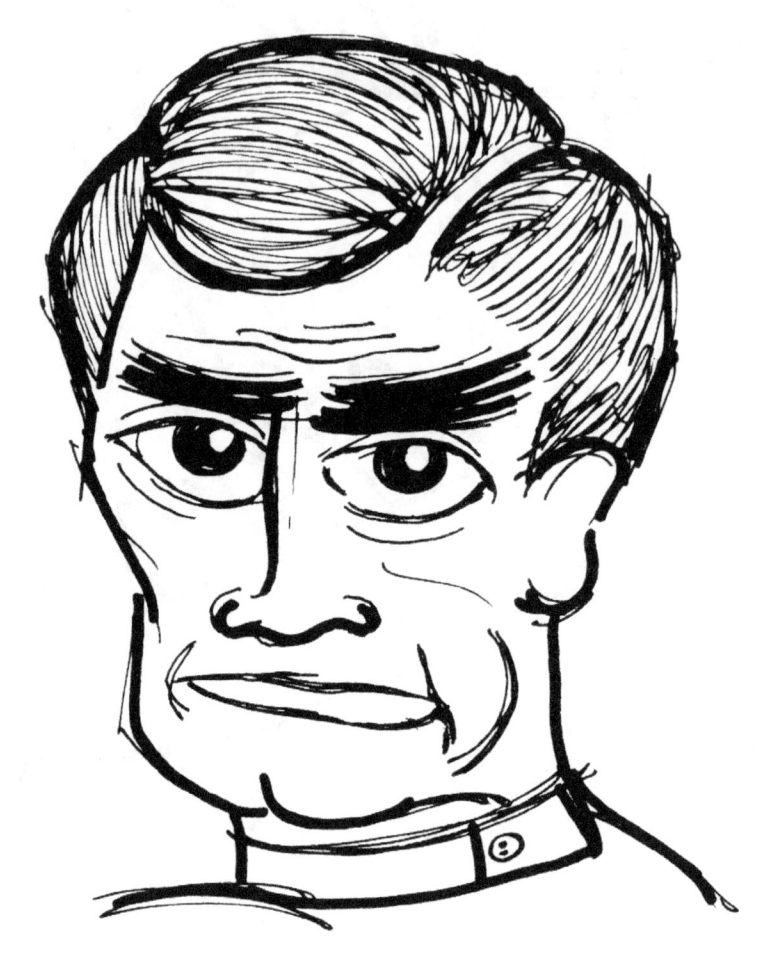

I AM THE GREAT **DR. ANTON PAZU** • THE OUT-
STANDING ORAL REHABILITATOR • I AM HAPPY!
I AM ENTHUSIASTIC • I AM A GREAT EXECUTIVE.
SOMETIMES I FEEL LIKE SAYING "THE HELL WITH IT"

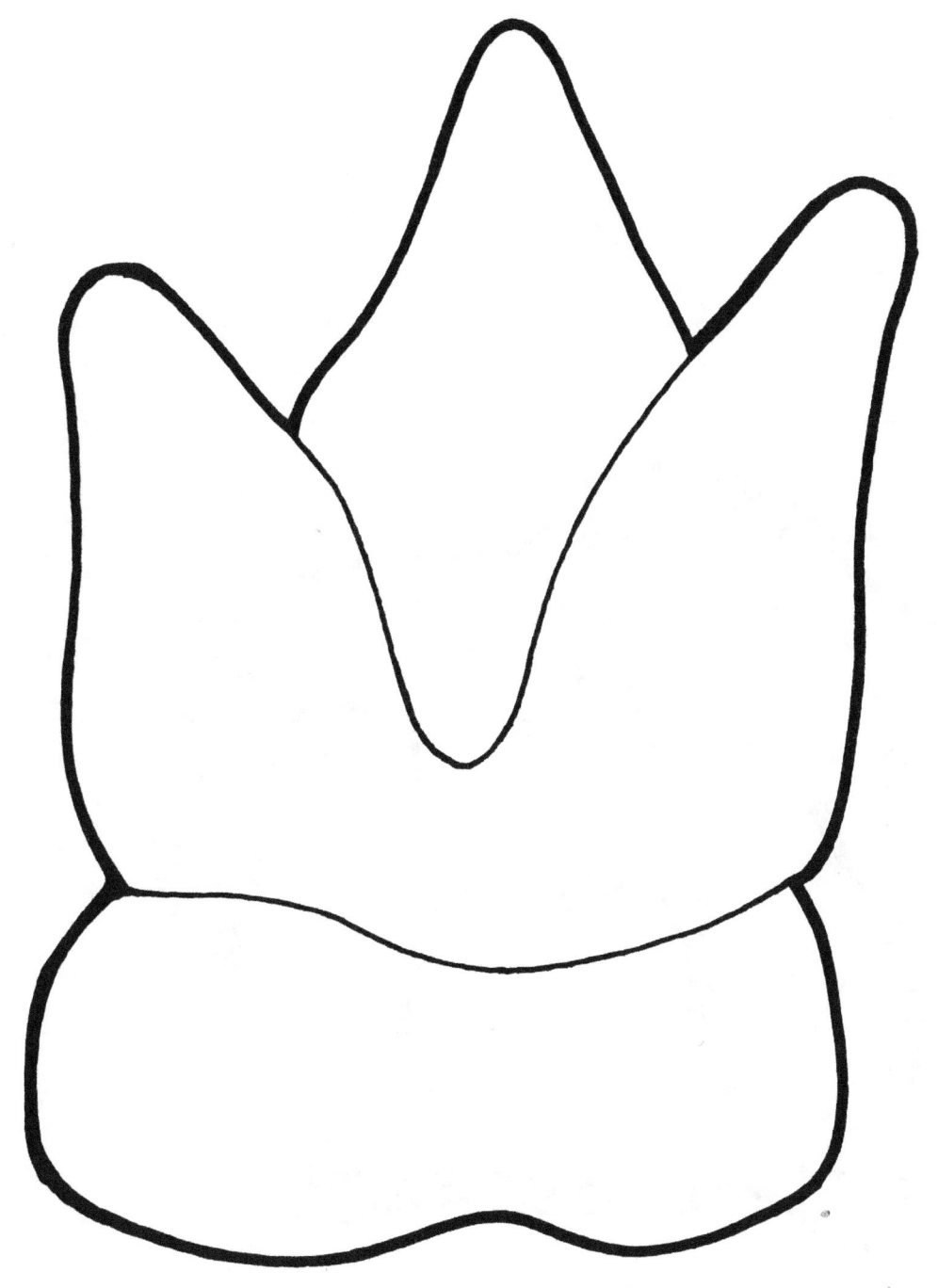

THIS IS A **TOOTH** • SOMETIMES I FIND IT
DIFFICULT TO EXTRACT BECAUSE THE ROOTS
ARE WRAPPED AROUND THE JAWBONE •••

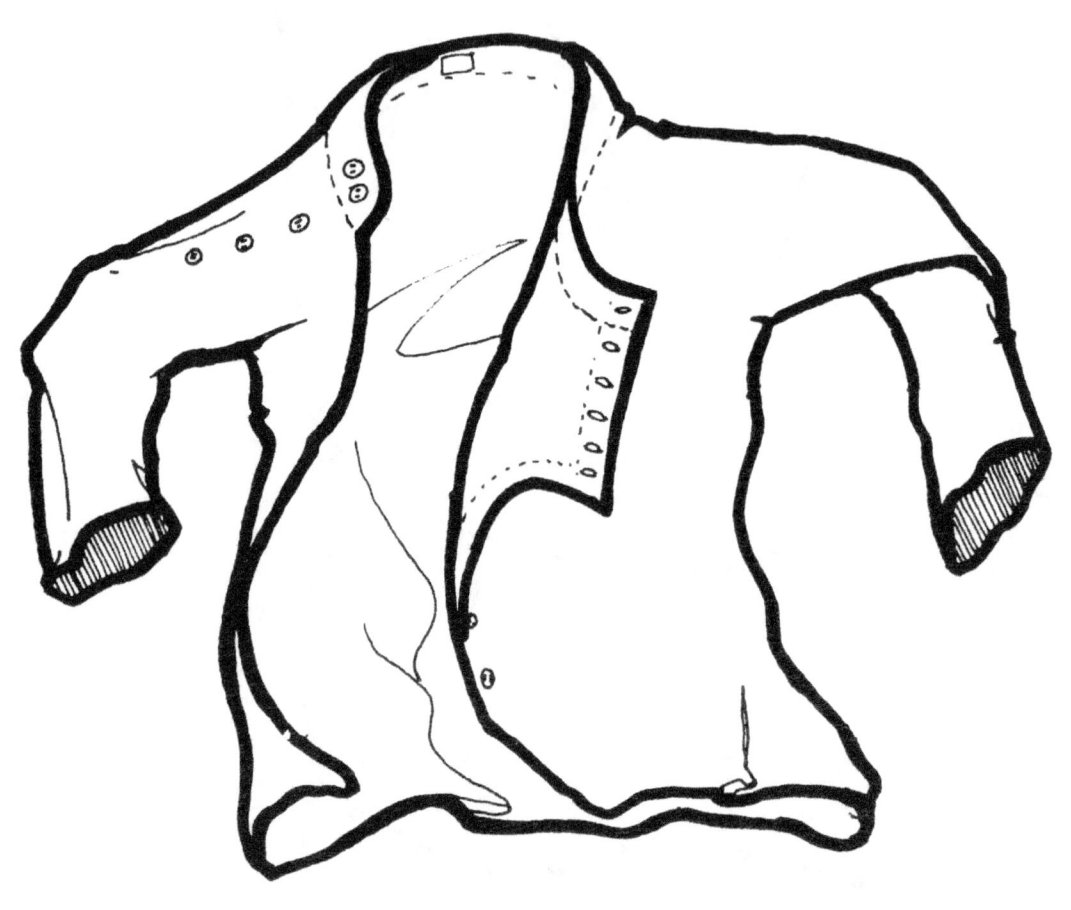

THIS IS MY SPARKLING WHITE **GOWN** • IT MAKES
ME STERILE...

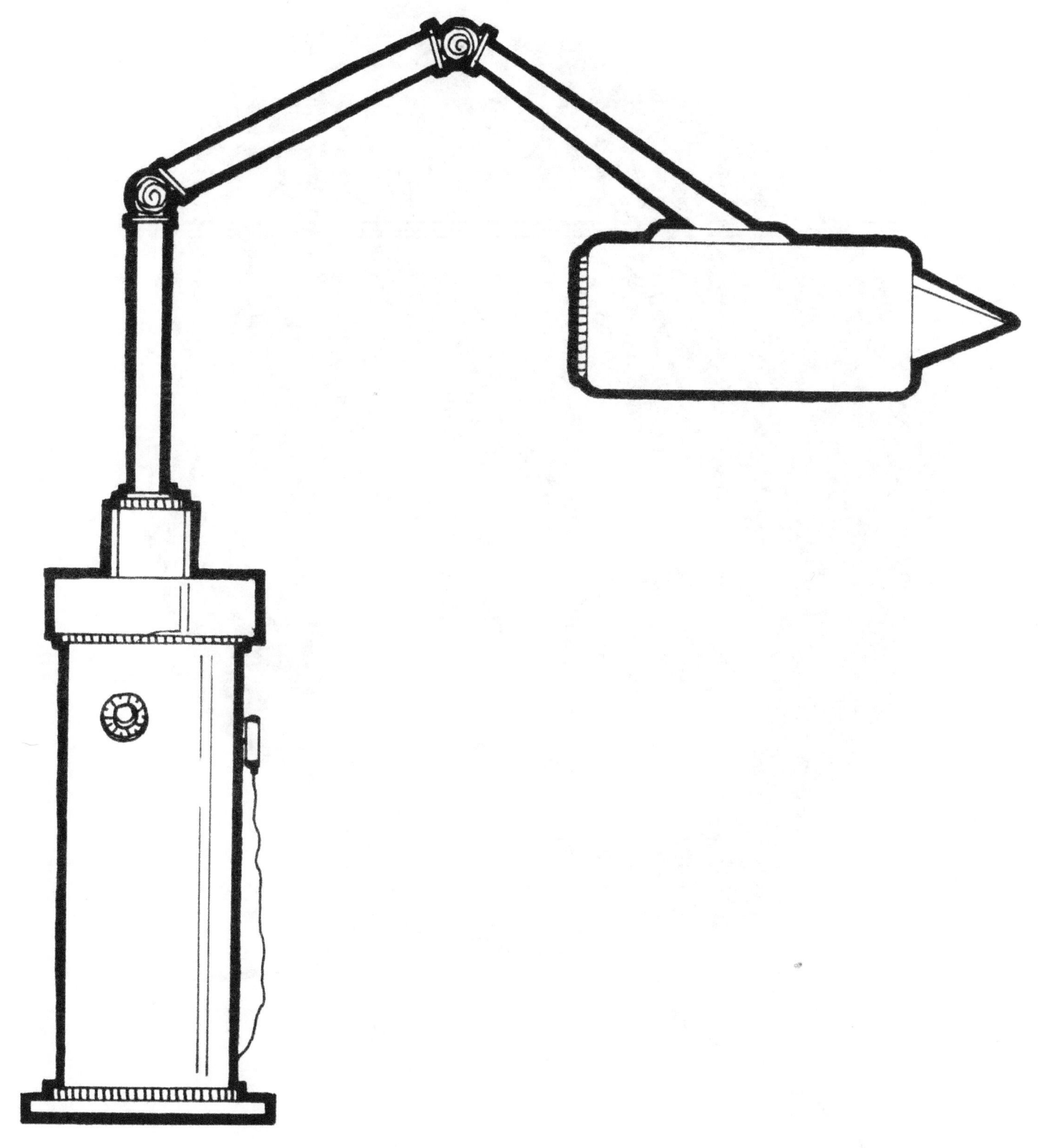

THIS DOES THE SAME THING !! ...

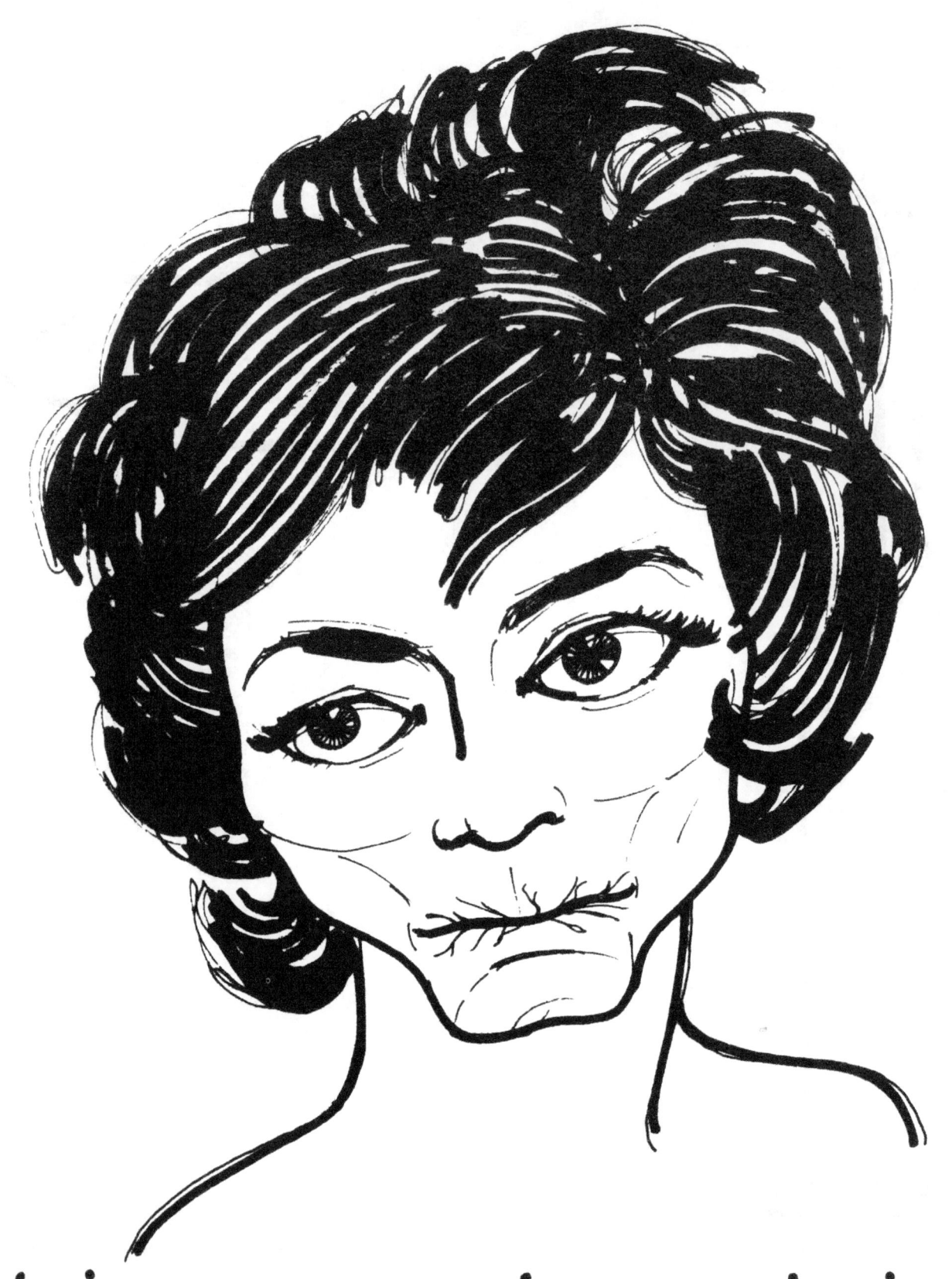

THIS IS A **DENTURE PATIENT** • SHE IS NINETEEN YEARS OLD • SHE IS HAPPY WHEN I TELL HER THAT NOW HER TROUBLES ARE OVER •••

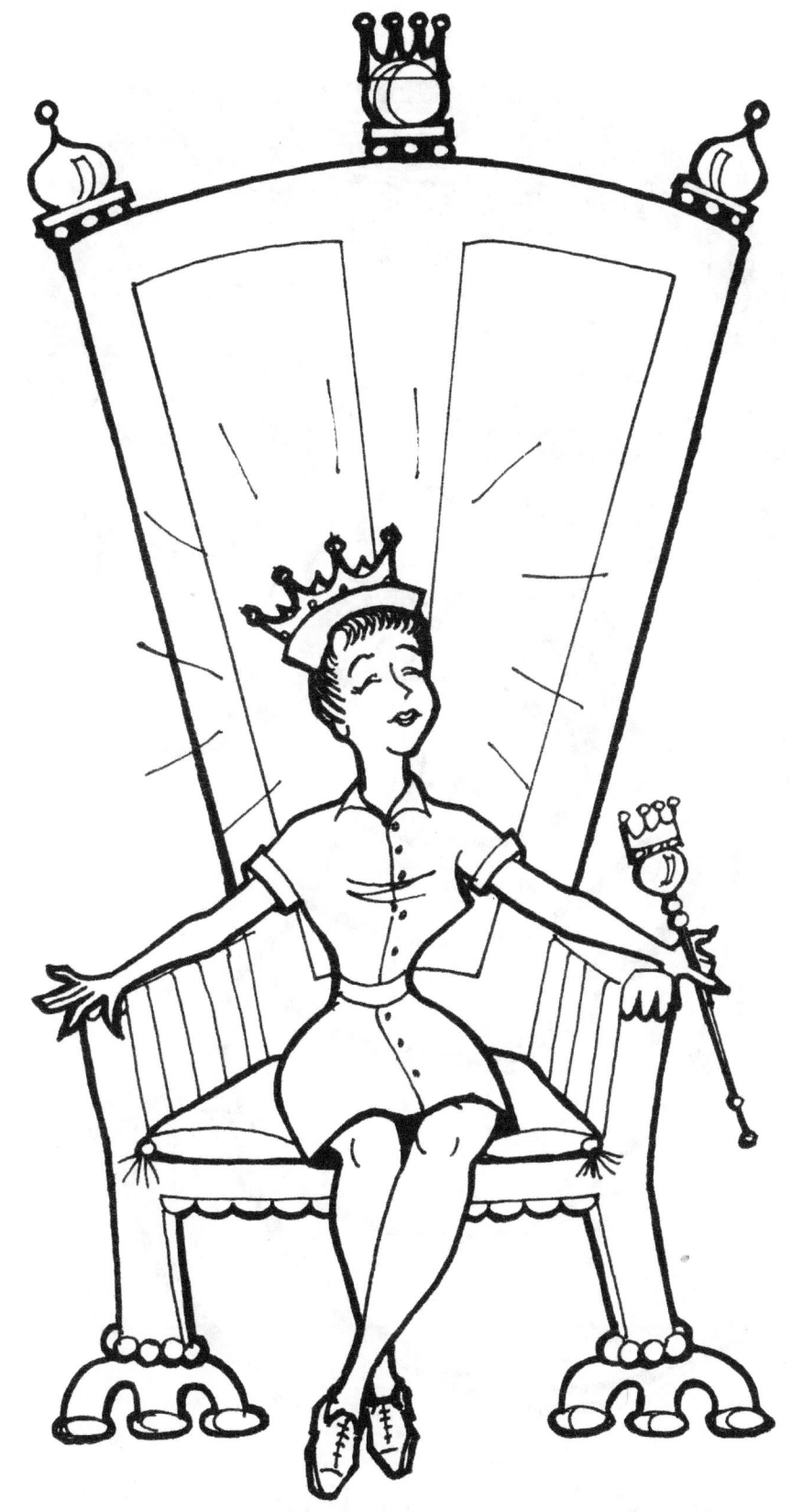

THIS IS MY **HYGIENIST**. SHE IS VERY INTELLIGENT.
SOMETIMES I FEEL INADEQUATE! ...

COLOR HER REGAL ...

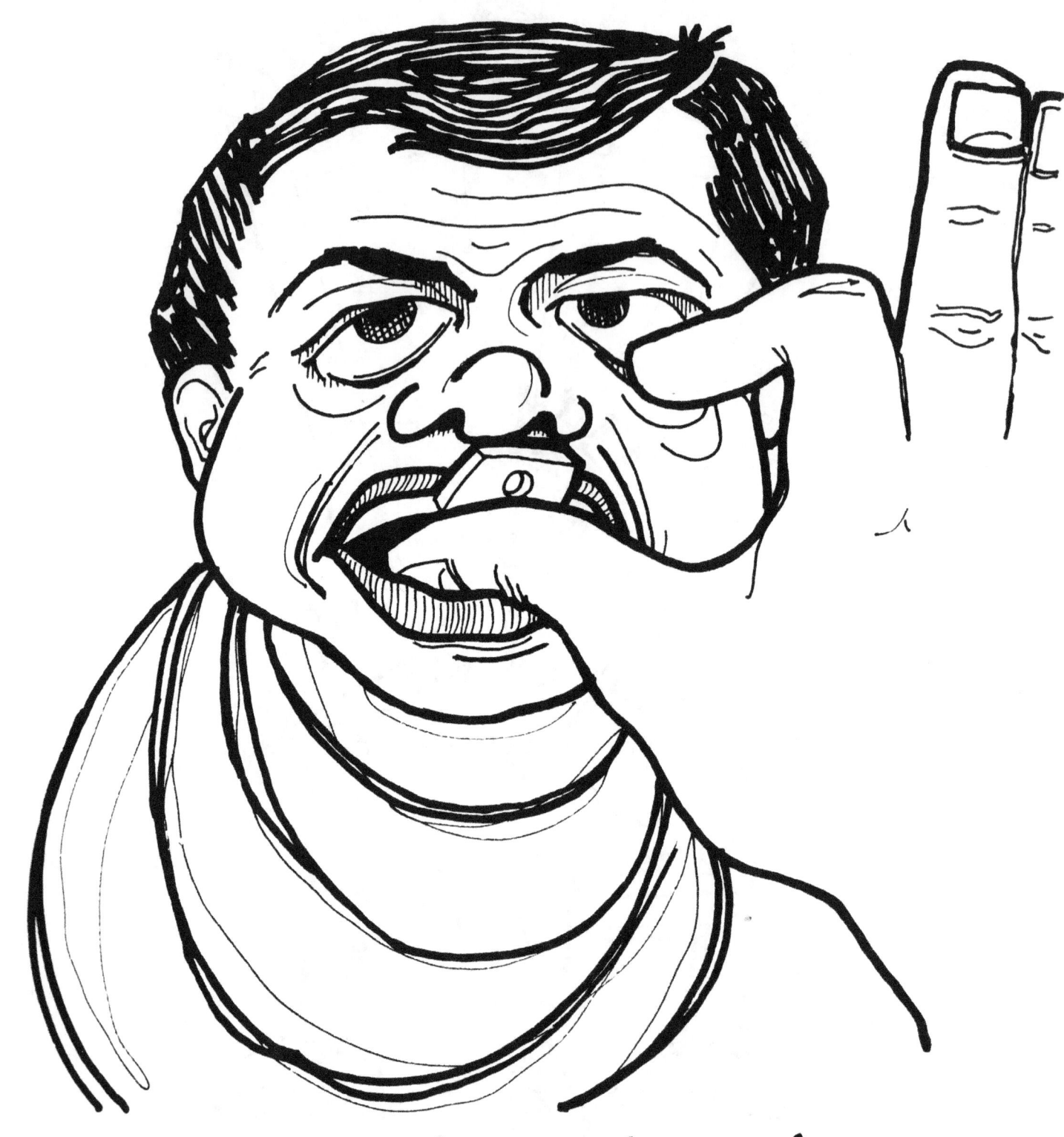

THIS IS MY THUMB • I AM TAKING AN IMPRESS-
ION • I FEEL IMPORTANT WHEN I AM TAKING
IMPRESSIONS •••

COLOR PATIENT GREEN •••

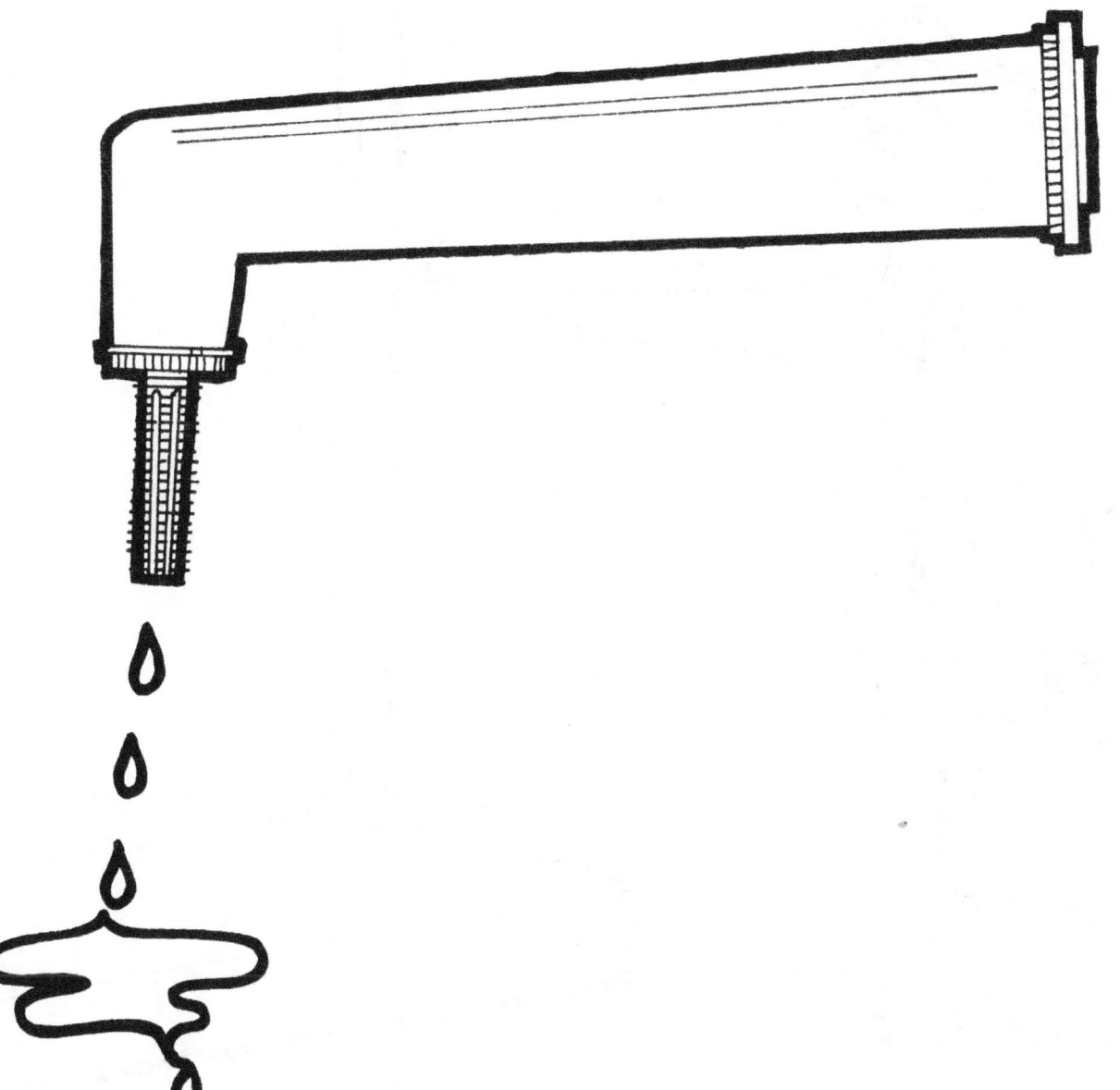

THIS IS MY **NEUTRON ROTOR**. IT REVOLVES AT 12 BILLION R.P.M. IT CUTS TEETH AND OTHER THINGS...

COLOR DROPS RED...

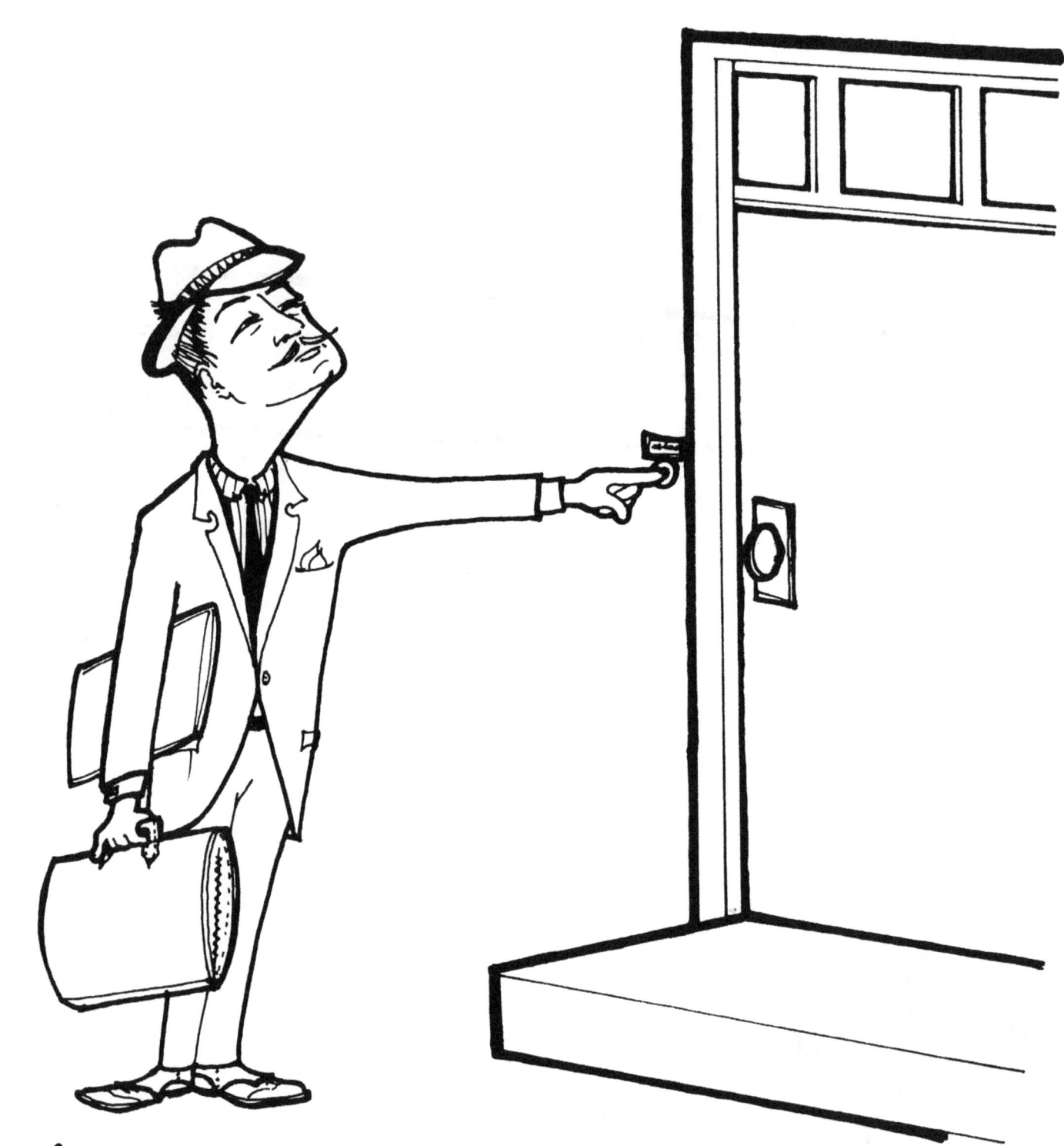

THIS IS MY **DENTAL SUPPLY SALESMAN** • HE
BRINGS ME THINGS • SOMETIMES I PAY HIM •
SOMETIMES I BUY THINGS I DON'T NEED ...
COLOR ME STUPID ON PAGE #4 ••

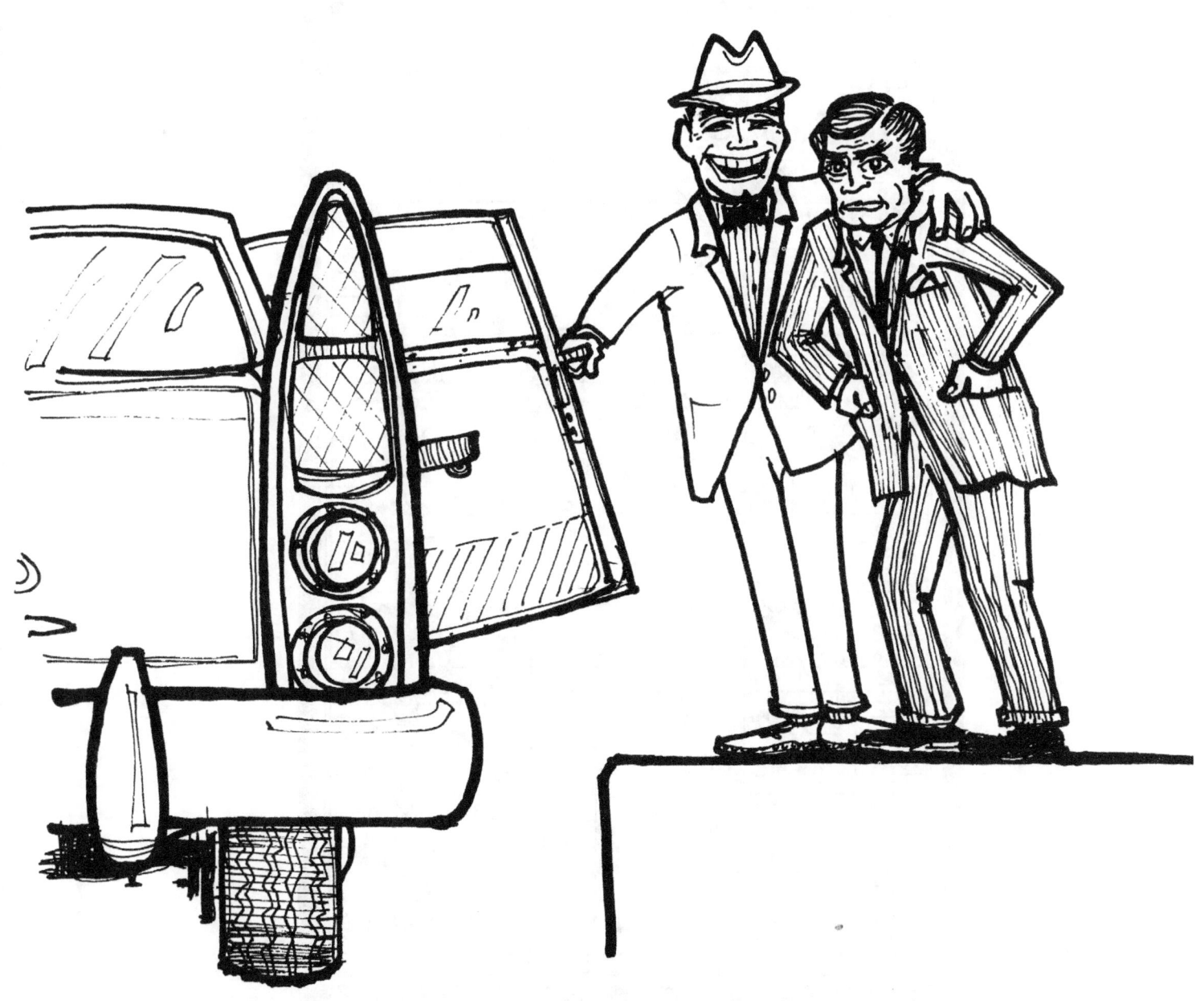

THIS IS AN **INSURANCE MAN** · TAKING ME TO LUNCH ·
WE TALK ABOUT MY FAMILY · HE TELLS ME THAT I
AM FAST BECOMING   KNOWN AS A VERY SUCCESSFUL
MAN · I LIKE HIM · I THINK HE LIKES ME · I AM
TAKING A PHYSICAL NEXT WEEK ···

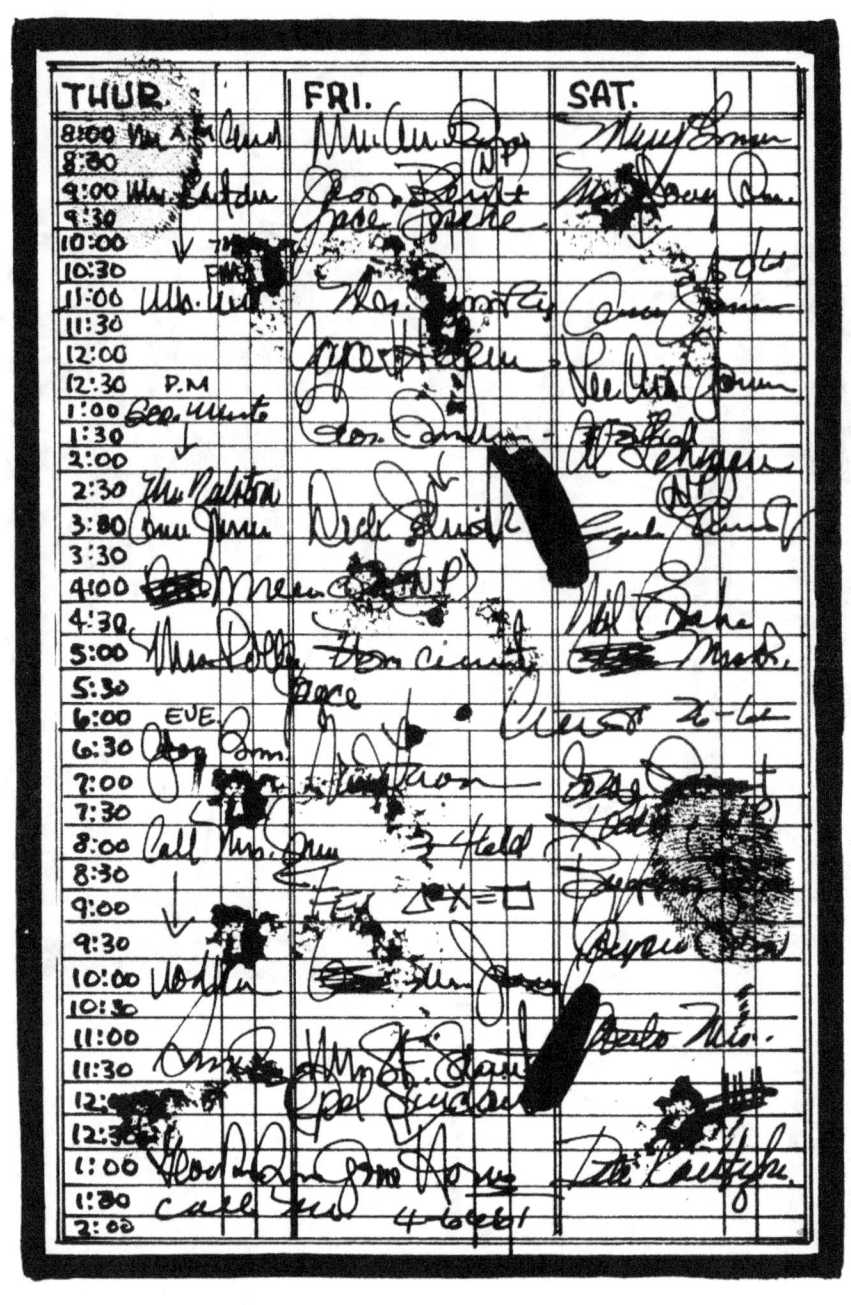

THIS IS MY **APPOINTMENT BOOK** · I MAKE ALL
APPOINTMENTS MYSELF · BECAUSE IT REQUIRES
AN ORGANIZED MIND ···

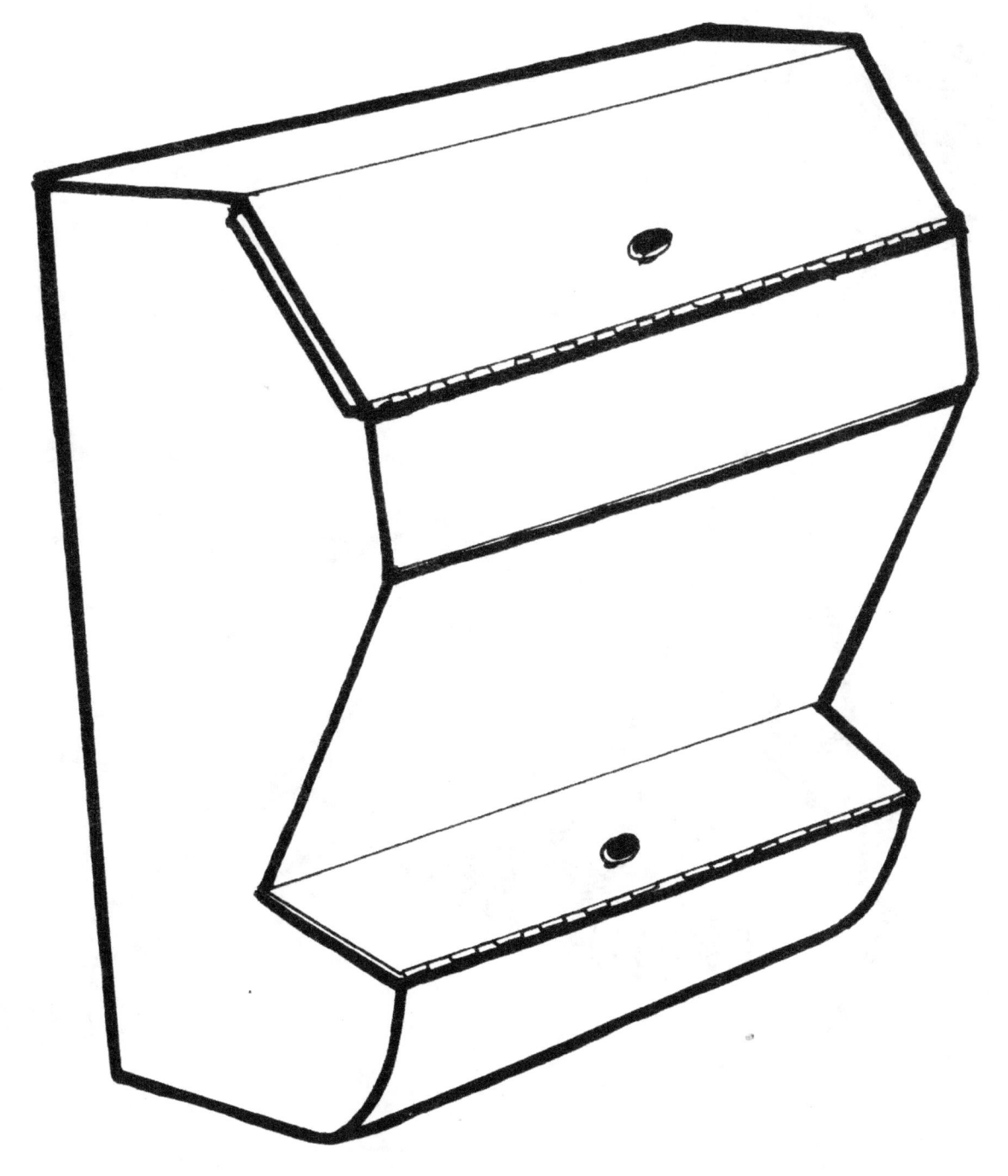

THIS IS MY SAFE • I KEEP MONEY AND OTHER
VALUABLES HERE • SOMETIMES PLASTER •••

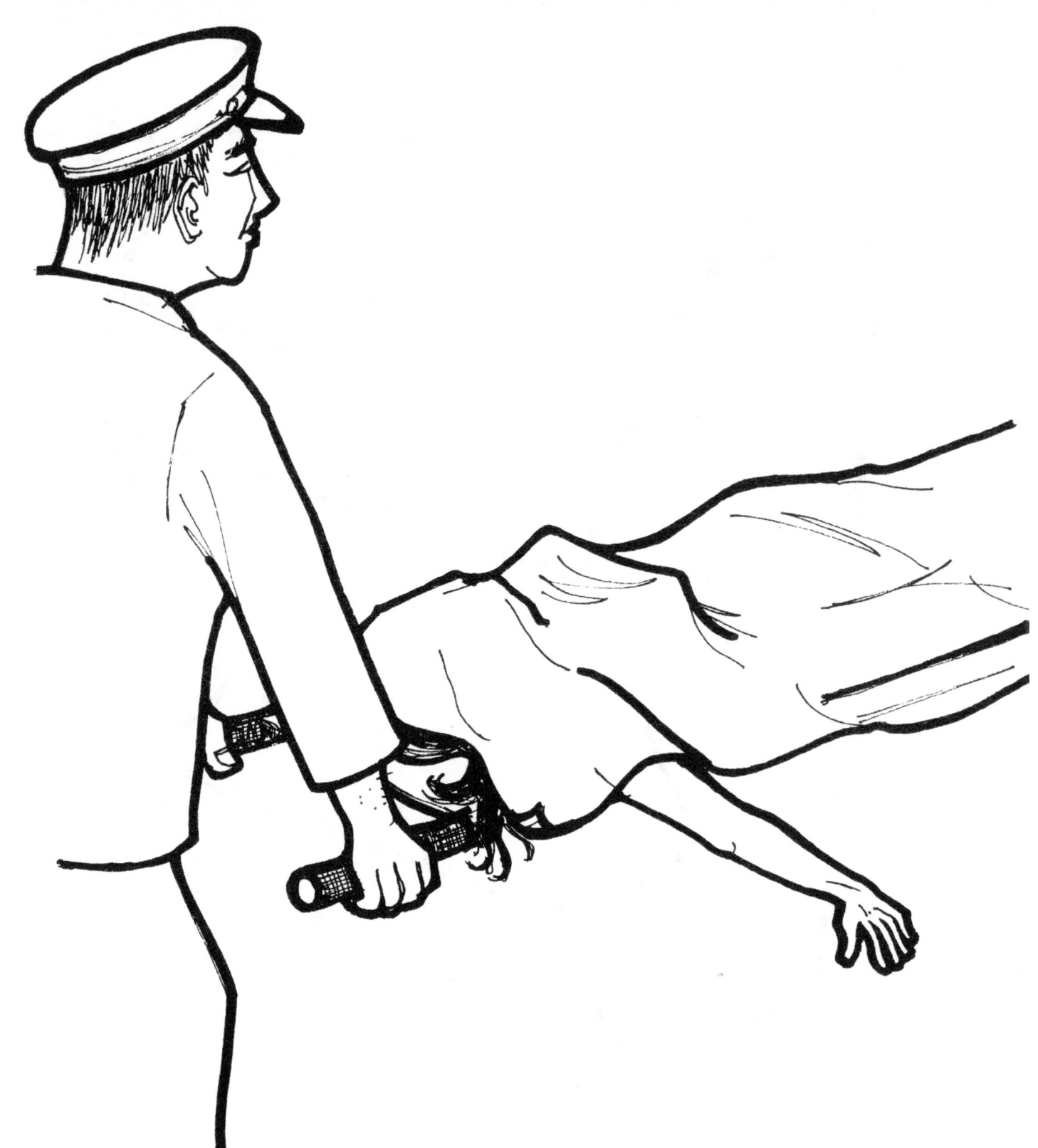

THIS IS MY FORMER ASSISTANT · I'LL NEVER FORGET HOW WELL SHE FIRED THE FURNACE AND SHOVELED THE WALK···

COLOR HER GRAY · VERY GRAY···

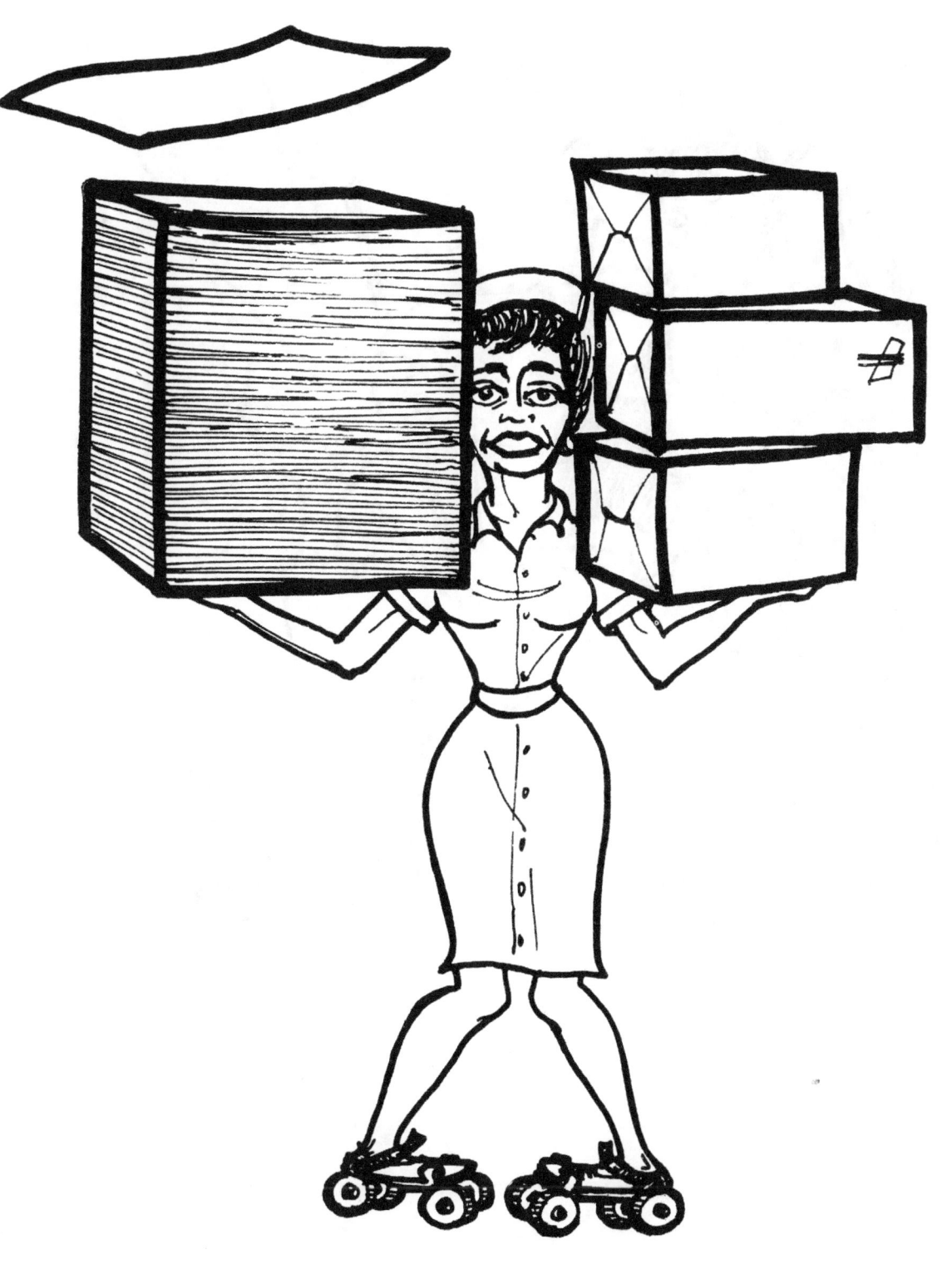

THIS IS MY PRESENT ASSISTANT. SHE WORKS
VERY HARD TOO. SOMEDAY I HOPE TO BE ABLE
TO PAY HER...

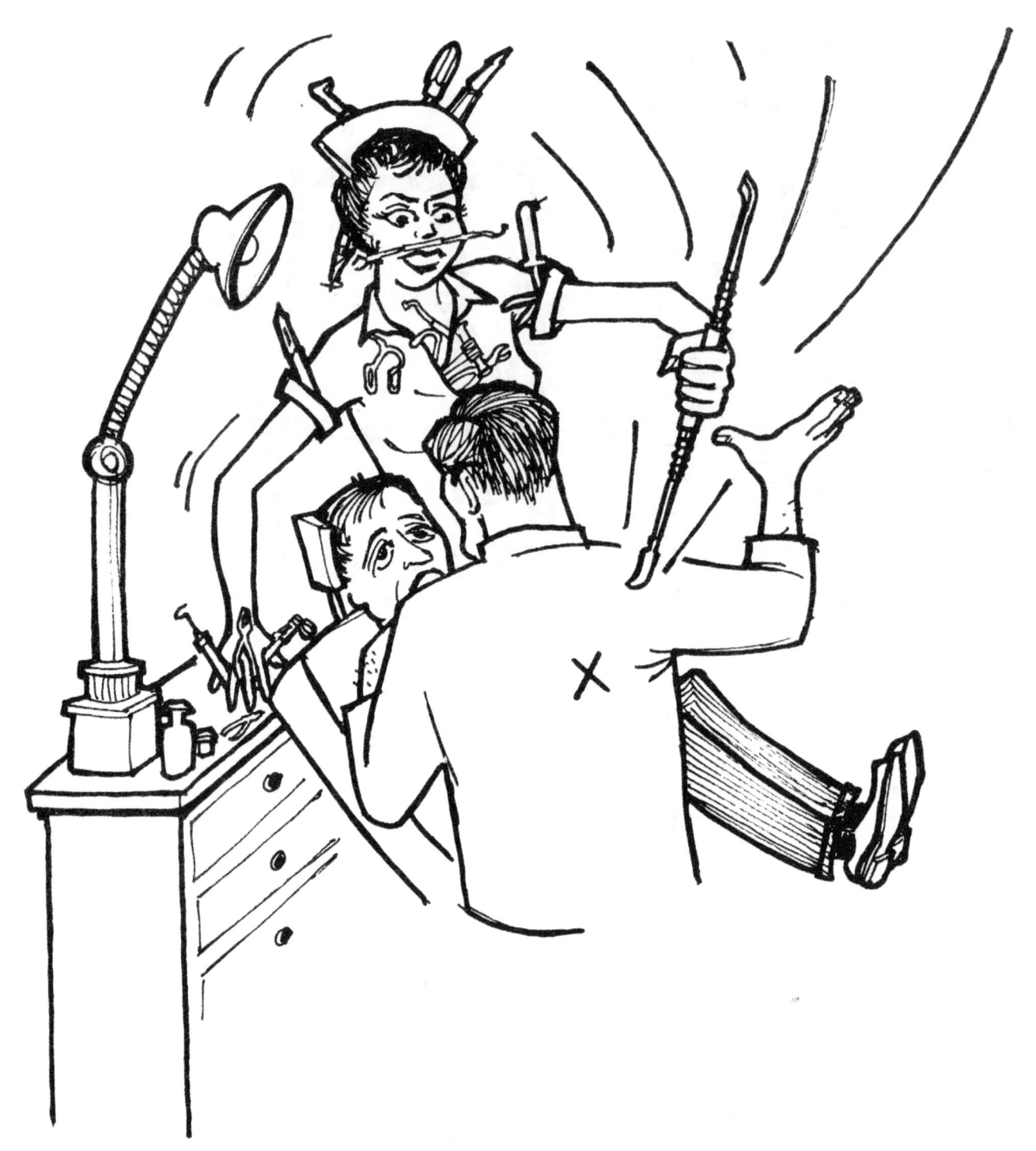

THIS IS MY **ASSISTANT AT THE CHAIR** · SOMETIMES
I THINK SHE GETS DISCOURGED ···
        COLOR CARVER STAINLESS ···

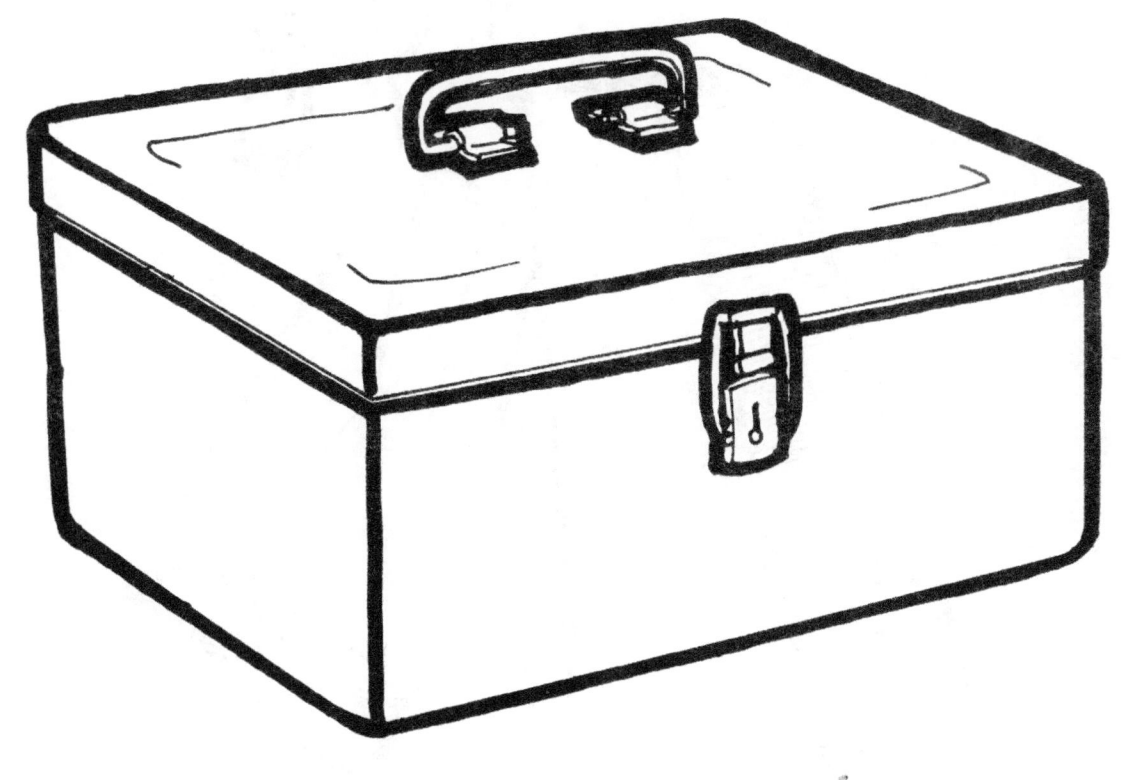

THIS IS MY ASSISTANTS PETTY CASH BOX • SOME-
TIMES IF I BORROW FROM IT - I GET MY
FINGERS SLAPPED •••

COLOR THEM RED •••

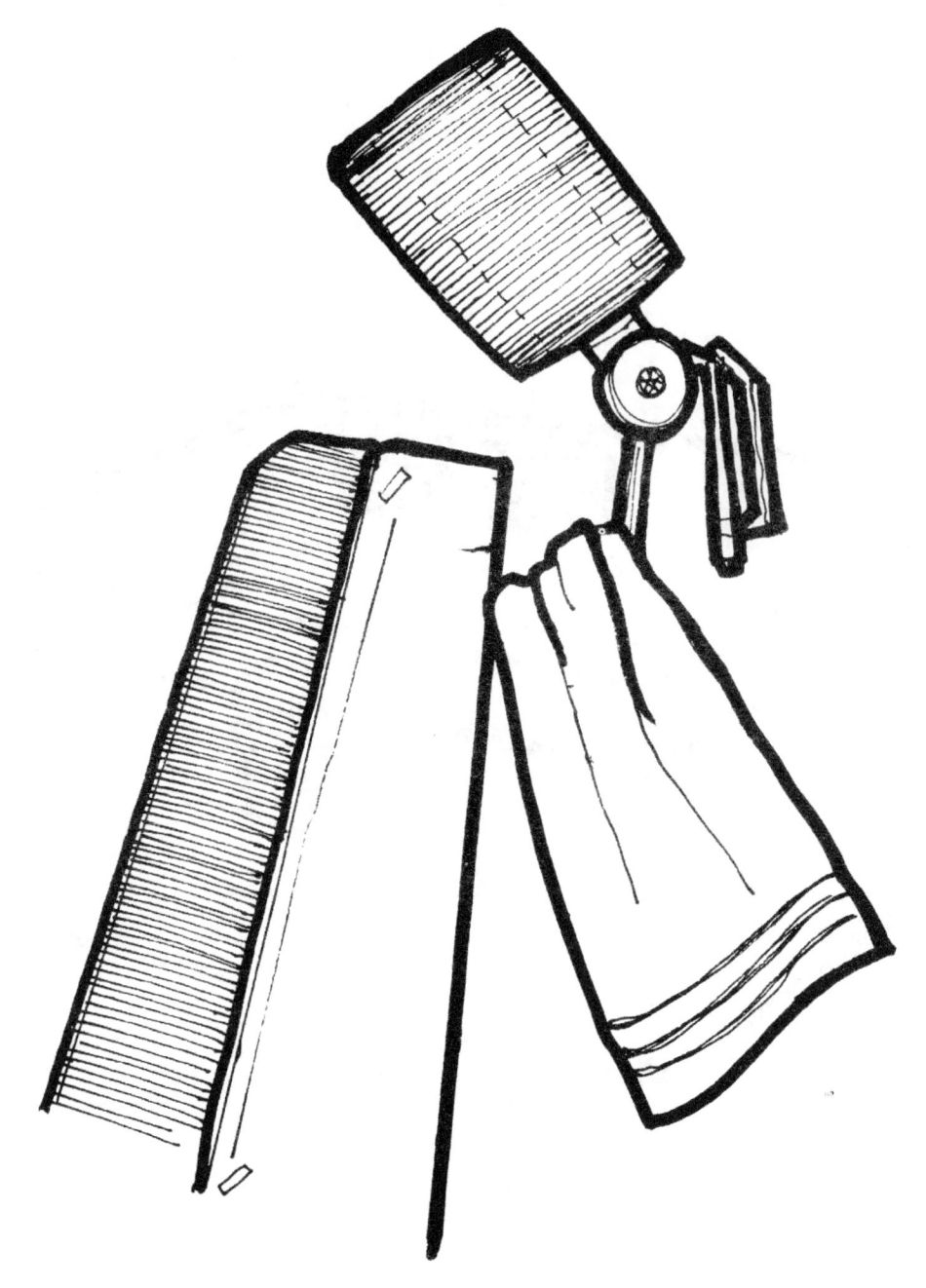

THIS IS A **TOWEL**• SOMETIMES I WIPE A CHILDS
CHIN WITH IT• SOMETIMES I--- WELL NEVER
MIND...

COLOR CHILD DEEP·PURPLE•

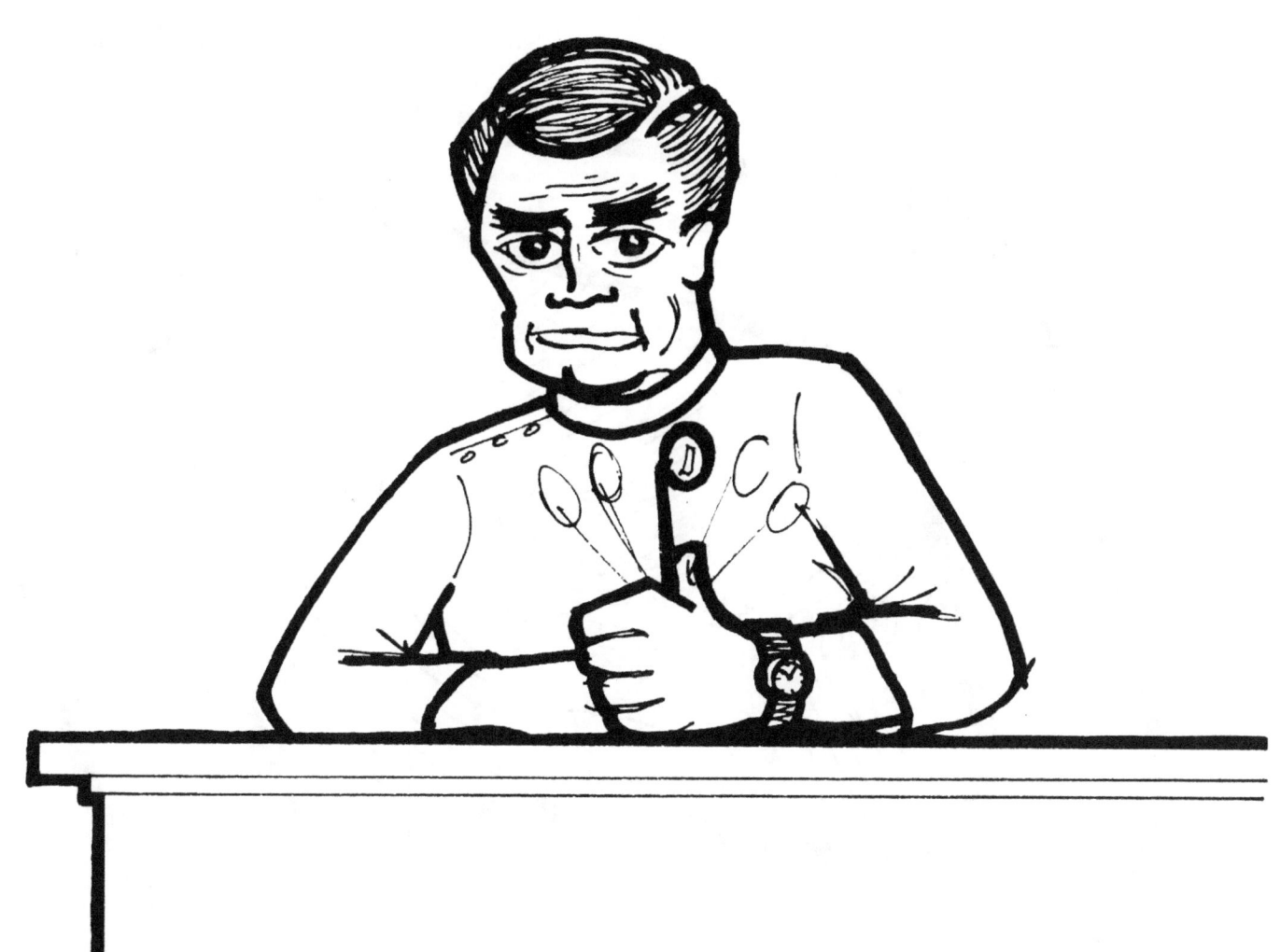

i HAVE A MASTERS DEGREE iN HUMAN RELATIONS.
i WiLL SHOW YOU HOW TO TAKE A DENTAL HiSTORY.
i AM SPEAKiNG TO THE PATIENT. i AM SAYiNG —
"i BELiEVE, MRS. JONES, THAT YOU ARE
JUSTiFiED iN PREFERRiNG CHiLDBiRTH*OVER
DENTiSTRY. THiNGS GET PRETTY ROUGH AROUND
HERE!"...

* iN THE FIELD OF SEMANTICS, iT iS MUCH MORE CULTURED TO SAY—
" CHiLD BiRTH" RATHER THAN "HAViNG A BABY"

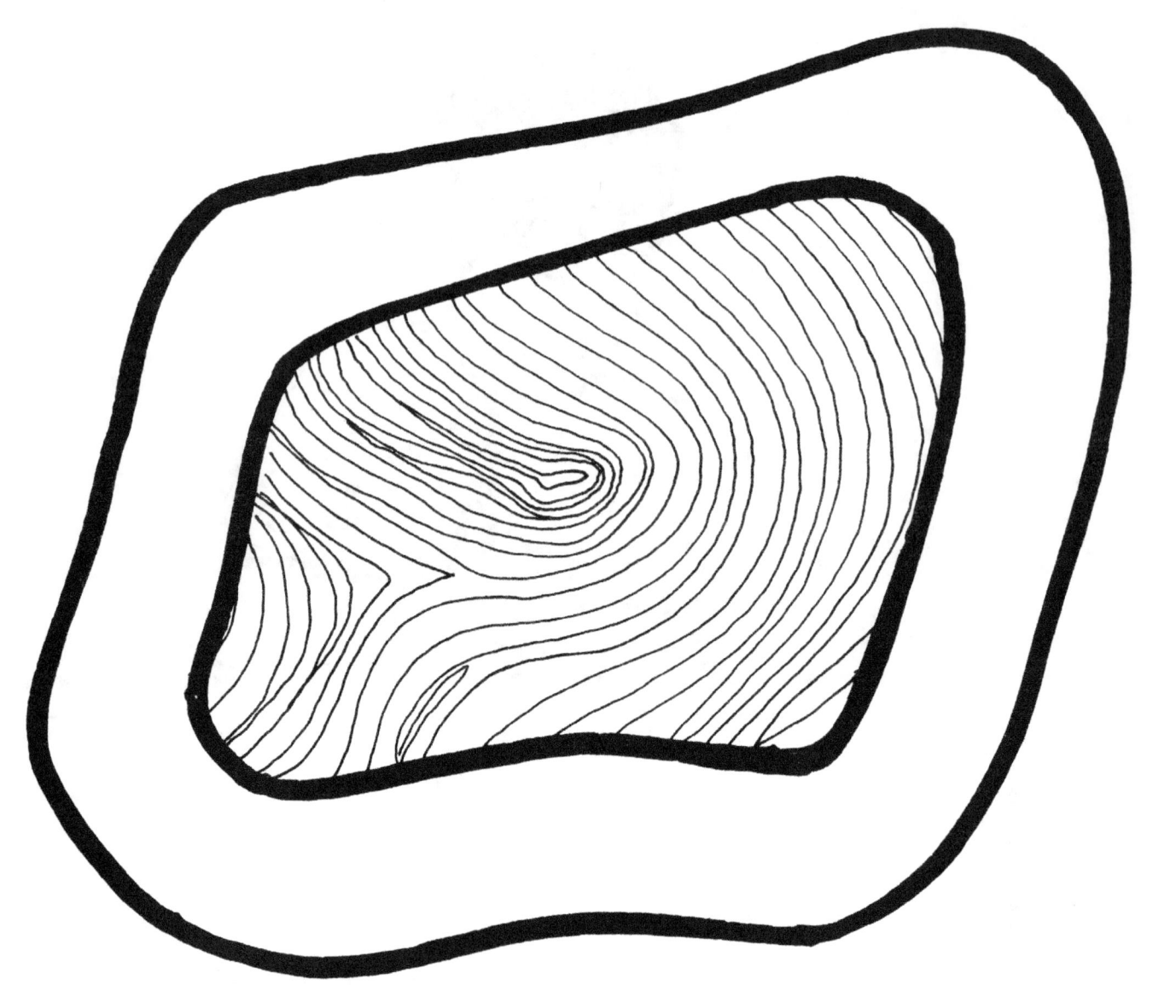

THIS IS SOME OF **MY WORK** · IT IS A PLATINUM
INLAY · WELL CONDENSED · AS YOU WILL NOTE I
AM A VERY PROUD OPERATOR····
COLOR INLAY SILVER·····

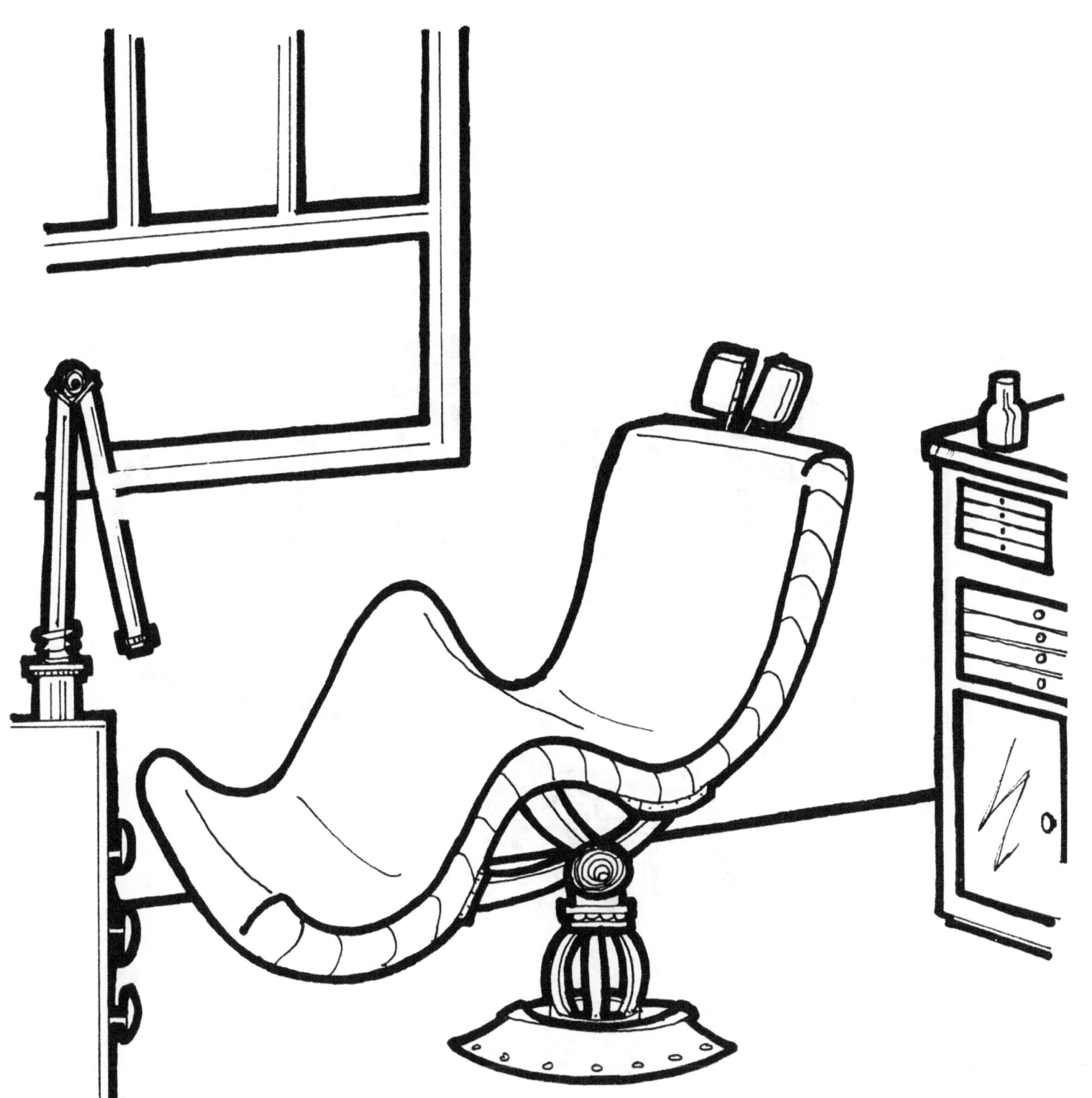

THIS IS MY NEW·CONTOUR CHAIR · SOME
PROCEDURES ARE VERY DIFFICULT WITH IT ·
i DON'T THINK i LIKE IT ···

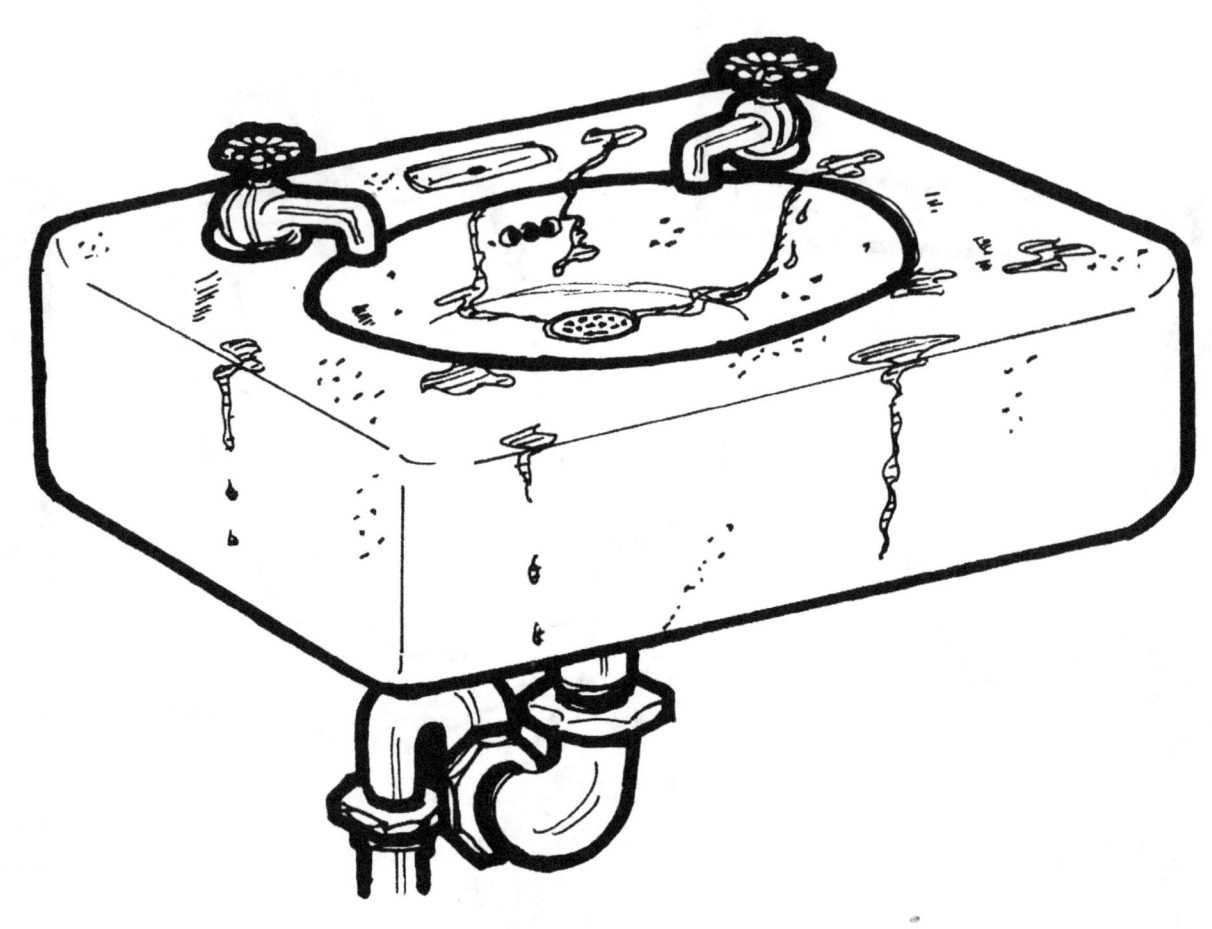

THIS IS MY **COMPOUND HEATER** · IT CAN BE USED
FOR OTHER THINGS TOO ...
COLOR IT SPECKLED BROWNISH WHITE·

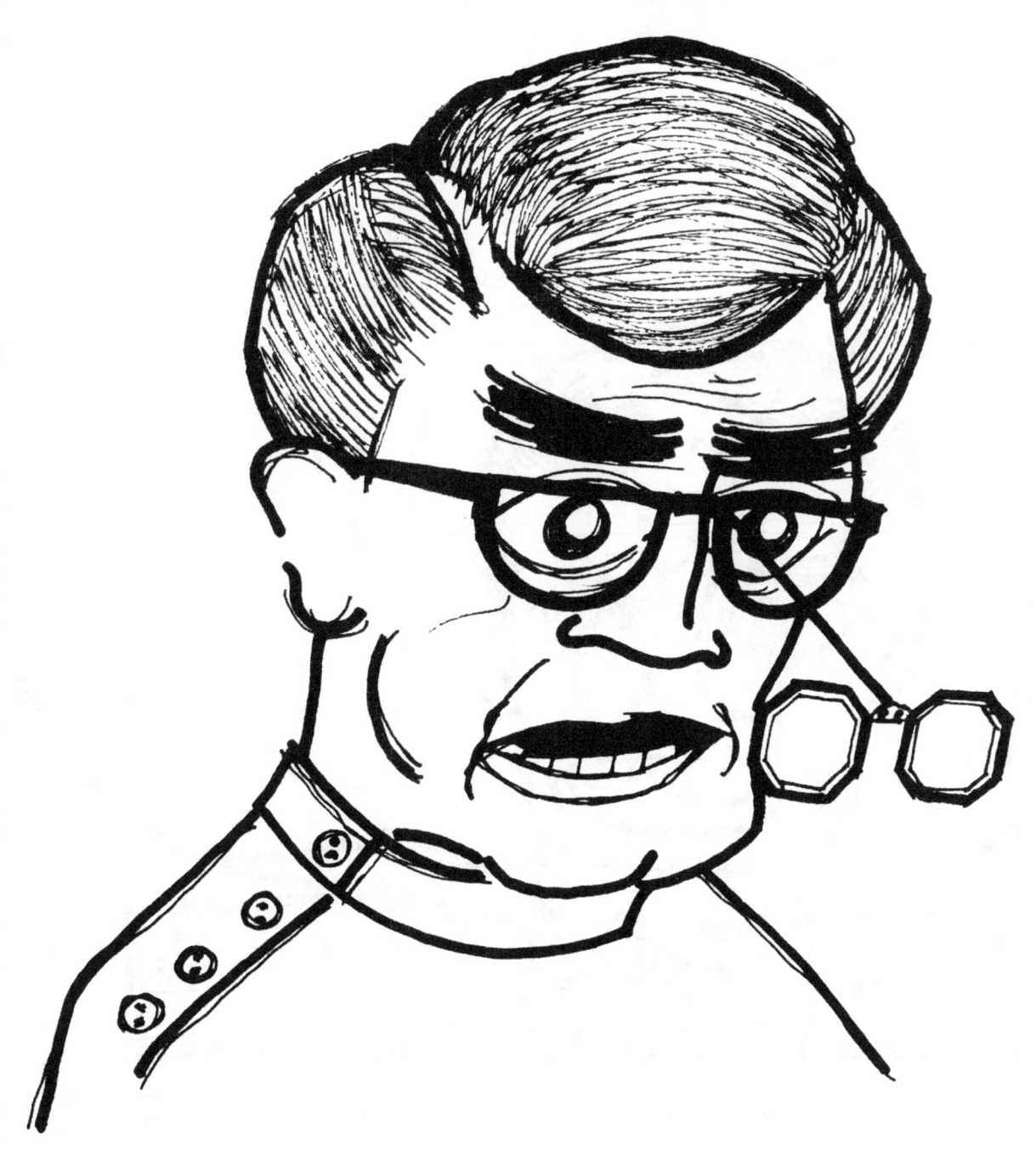

THIS IS **ME** AT THE CHAIR • I AM SAYING •
"MY GOD; MRS. BROWN, YOU'RE RIGHT!
THERE IS NOTHING LEFT!"

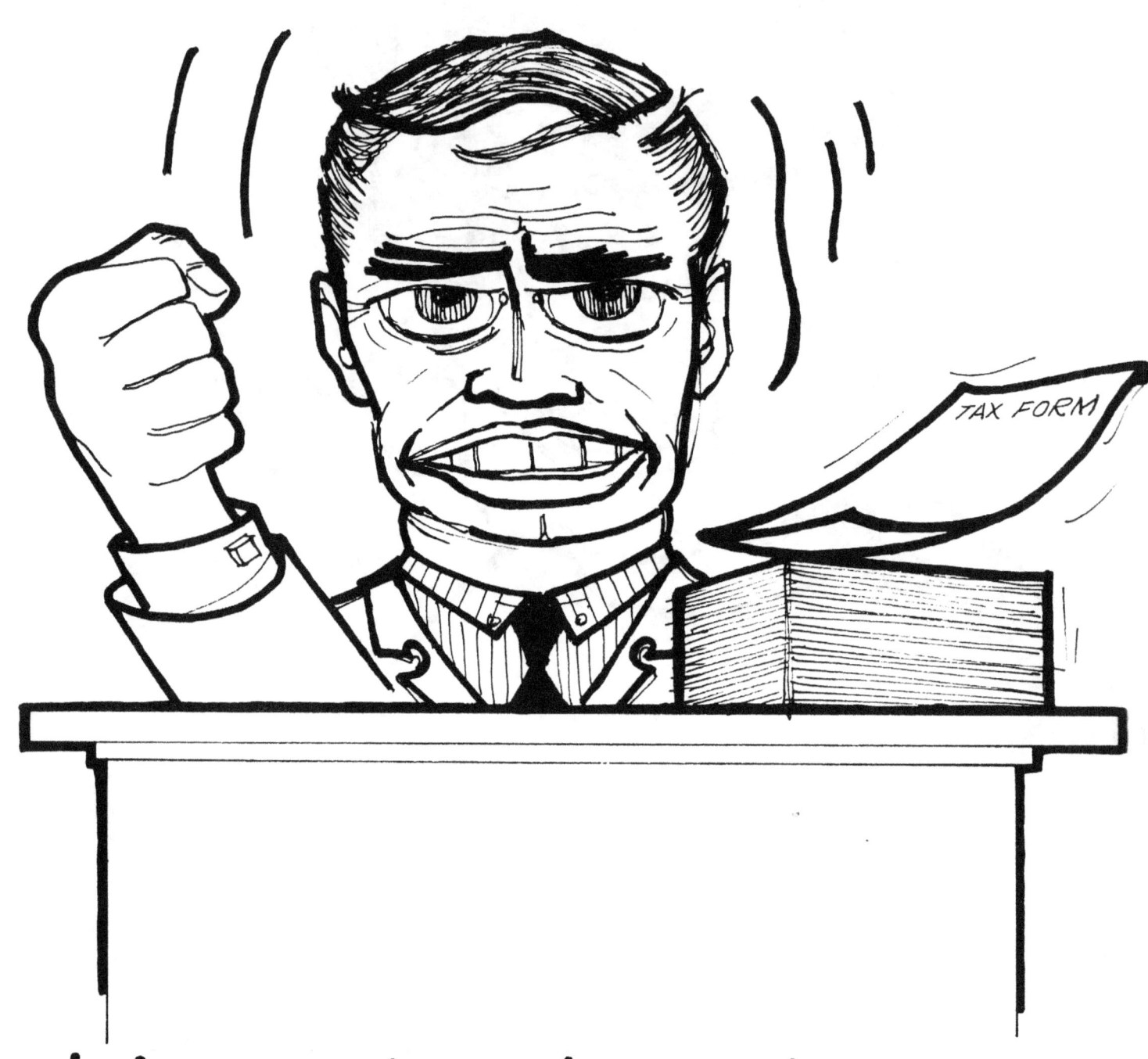

THIS IS MY **AUDITOR** . I HATE HIM . MY CAR
IS 100% DEDUCTIBLE . WHY DOES HE ALWAYS
ARGUE ? ...

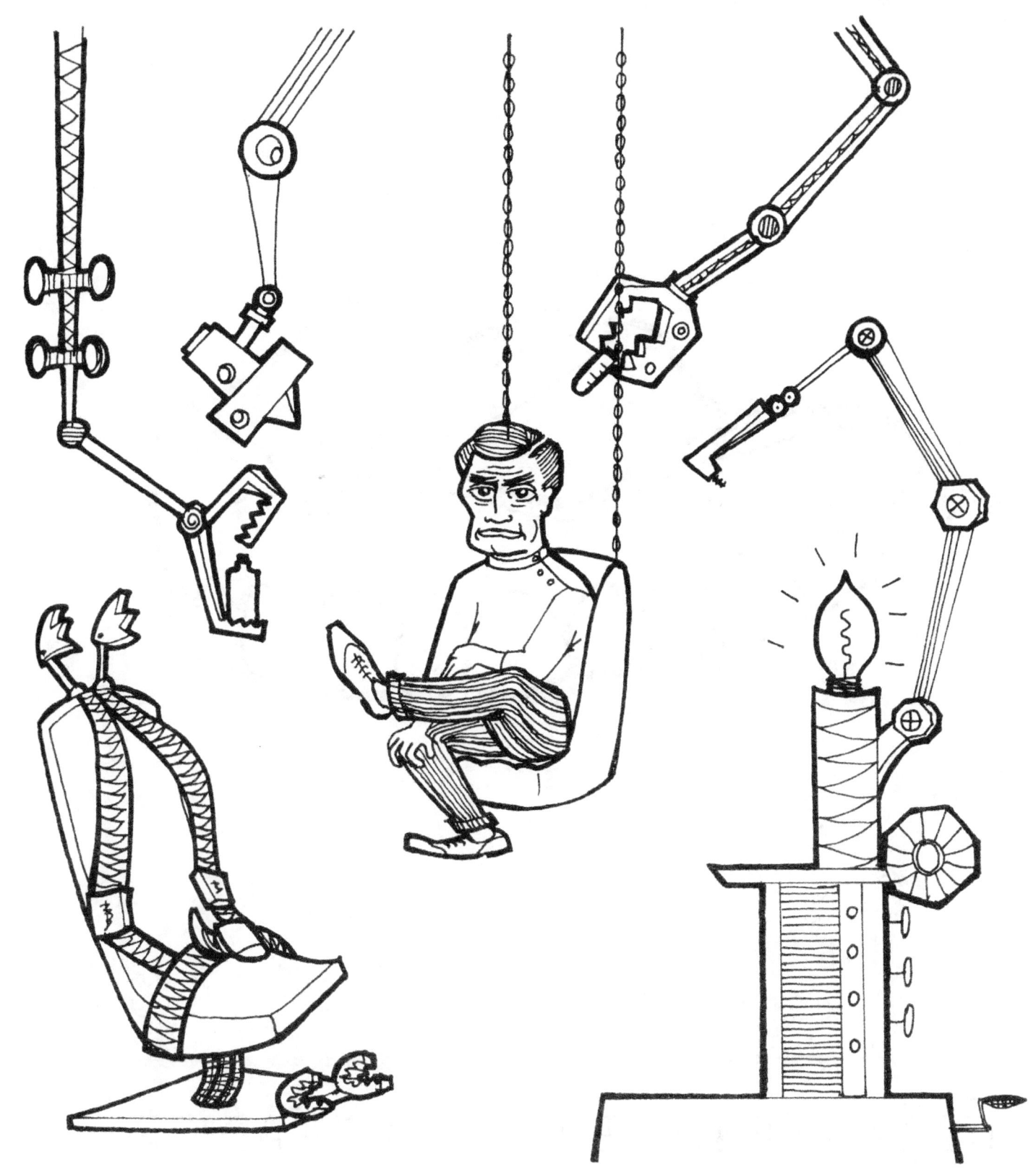

THIS IS ME LOOKING AT NEW EQUIPMENT • I GET VERY EXCITED • I PREFER A BUCKET SEAT OVER A STOOL BECAUSE YOU CAN HANG IT FROM THE CEILING • COLOR ME CONFUSED •••

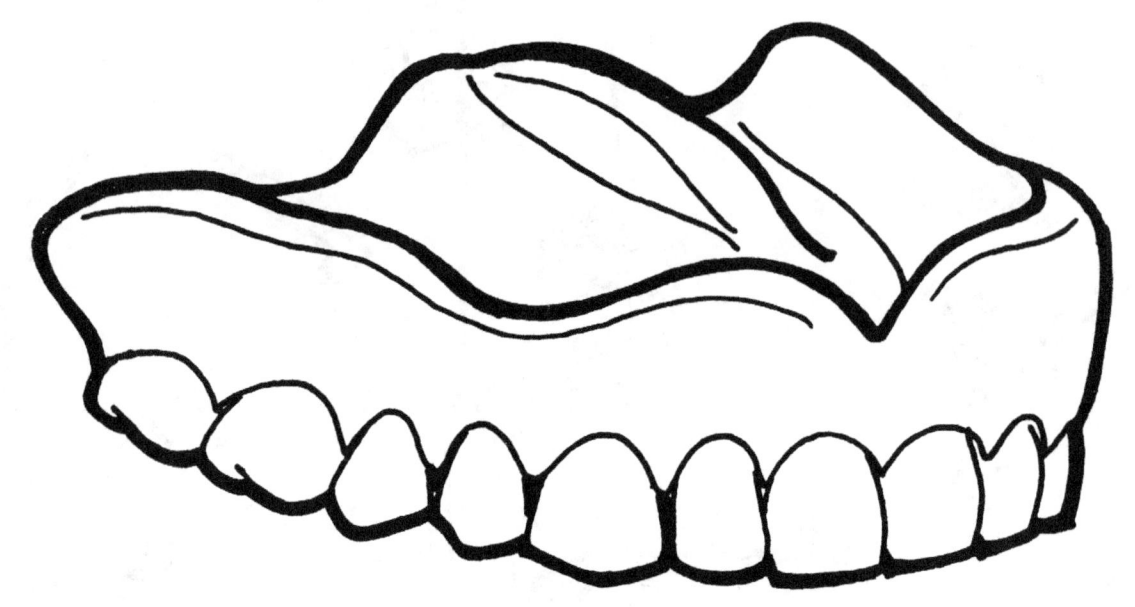

THIS IS A **DENTURE** • IT HAS HAD 732 ADJUSTMENTS • I WONDER IF THE PATIENT REALIZES HOW HAPPY I AM TO BE OF SUCH EXTREME SERVICE •••

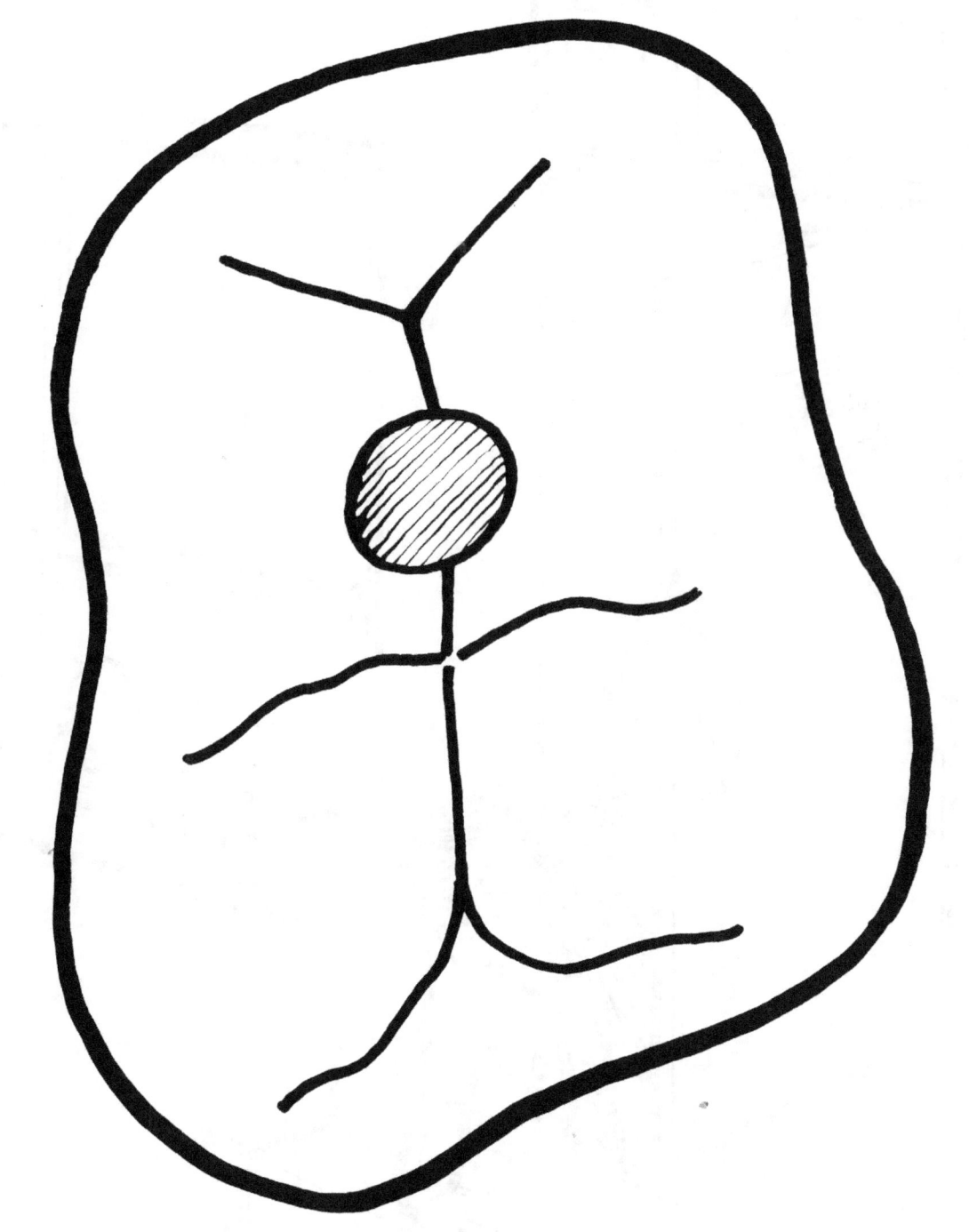

THIS IS A **PATIENT** WHOSE FILLING FELL OUT· I EXPLAIN TO HER THAT SHE HAS A PROBLEM· THAT HER TEETH ARE SOFT AND WILL NOT HOLD FILLINGS· SHE UNDERSTANDS···

COLOR HOLE SOFT···

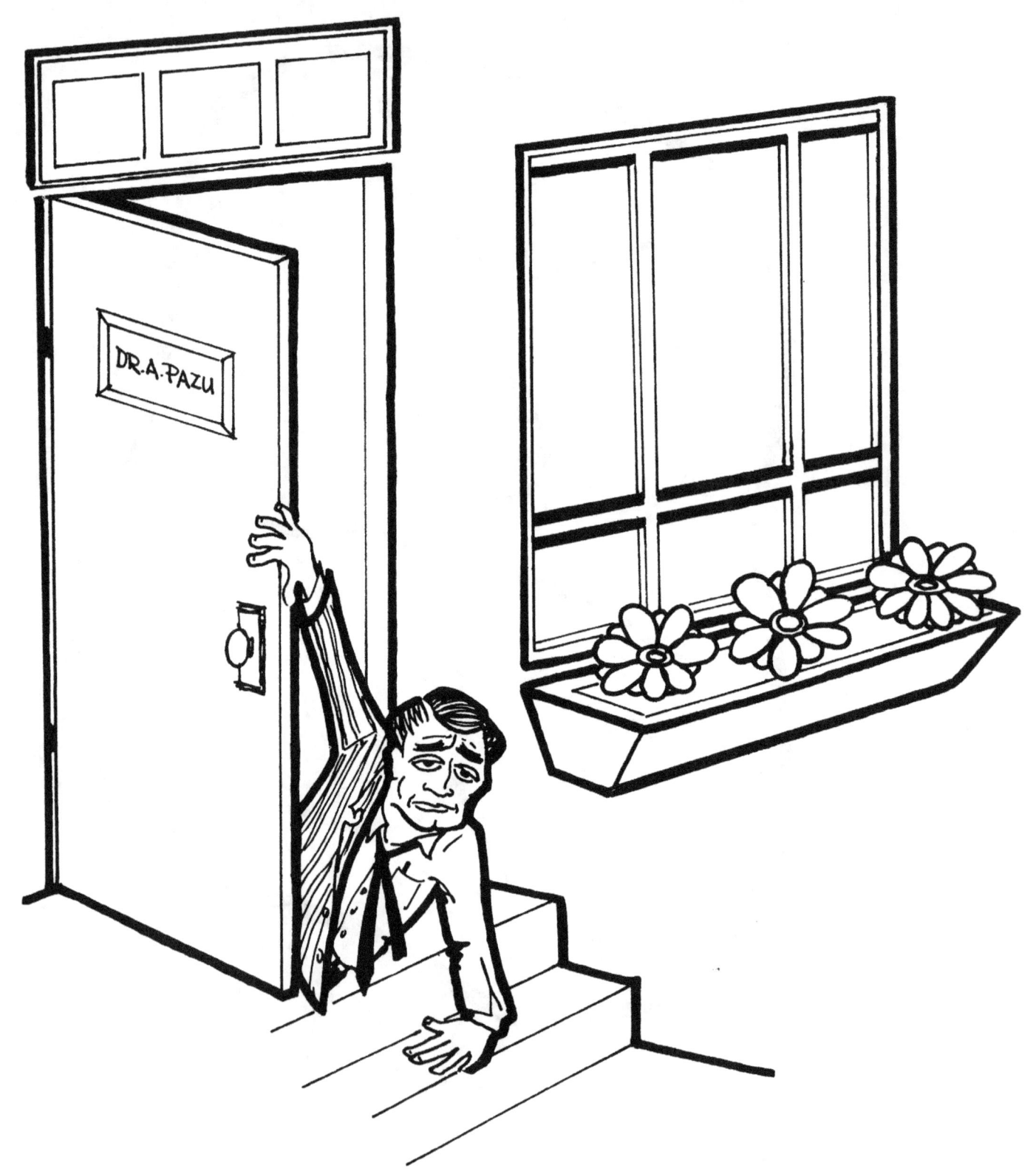

THIS IS ME. LEAVING THE OFFICE, PROMPTLY AT 11 P.M. MY STAFF LEFT SIX HOURS AGO. BUT THEY ARE NOT AS STRONG AS THE GREAT ANTON PAZU. I UNDERSTAND····

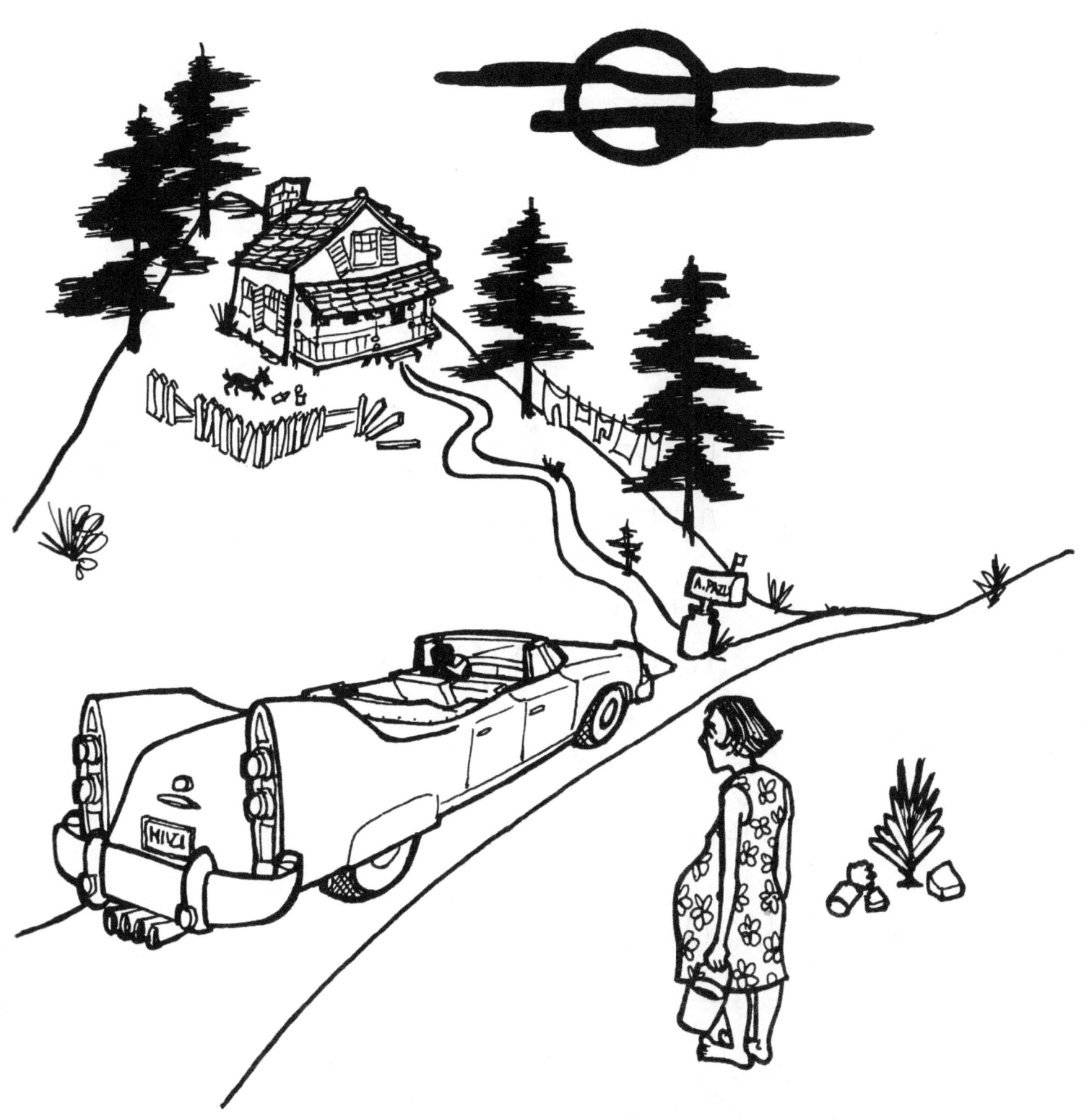

THIS IS ME • ARRIVING HOME • MY CHILDREN
ALWAYS WANTED A CONVERTIBLE • YOU WILL
NOTE • I TRY TO SATISFY MY FAMILY •••
COLOR CONVERTIBLE EXPENSIVE •

AND FINALLY:

IF YOU SHOULD EVER WISH TO VISIT MY OFFICE.
PLEASE WRITE AHEAD. BECAUSE I AM
CONTEMPLATING A MOVE. THINGS ARE NOT
EXACTLY THE WAY I WANT THEM IN MY
PRESENT LOCATION.

THIS IS A LOUSY TOWN..

SINCERELY YOURS,

Dr. Anton Pazu

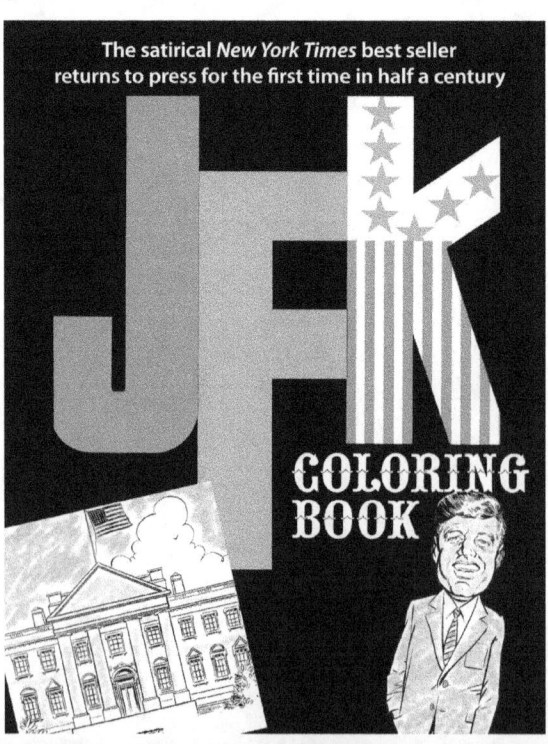

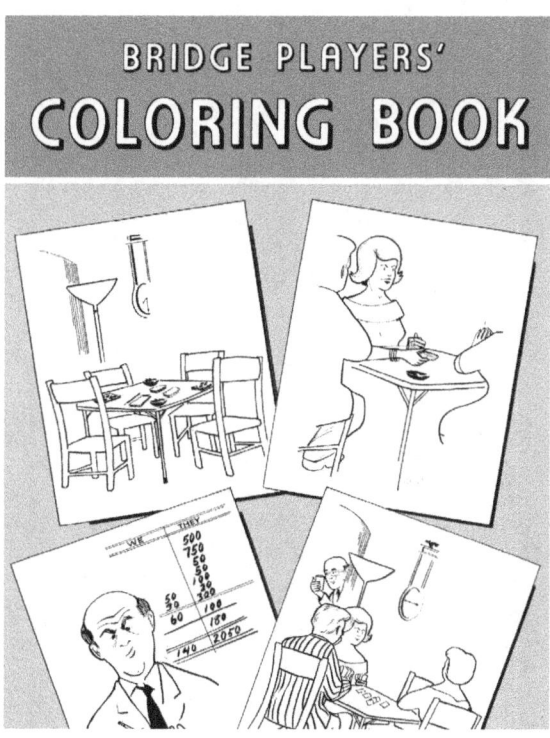

www.ingramcontent.com/pod-product-compliance
Lightning Source LLC
Chambersburg PA
CBHW080644190526
45169CB00009B/3501